PURPLE HEARTS

based on the novel
How Can You Mend This Purple Heart
by
Terry L. Gould

adapted for stage
and readers theater by
Terry L. Gould and M.C. Nelson

To contact Terry Gould,
email:
purplescribe68@gmail.com

***Ideas into Books*®**
W E S T V I E W
P.O. Box 605
Kingston Springs, TN 37082
www.publishedbywestview.com

PURPLE HEARTS
a stage play adaptation of *How Can You Mend This Purple Heart*
by Terry L. Gould

This book is a work of fiction. Names, characters, places and incidents either are products of the author's imagination or are used fictitiously. Any resemblance to actual events or locales or persons, living or dead, is entirely coincidental.

Copyright © 2025 Terry L. Gould and M.C. Nelson
All rights reserved, including the right to reproduction, storage, transmittal, or retrieval, in whole or in part in any form.

ISBN 978-1-62880-680-9

First edition: Memorial Day 2025

Good faith efforts have been made to trace copyrights on materials included in this publication. If any copyrighted material has been included without permission and due acknowledgment, proper credit will be inserted in future printings after notice has been received.

Digitally printed worldwide on acid free paper.

PURPLE HEARTS
STAGE PLAY
CHARACTER DESCRIPTIONS
In Order of Appearance

"Doc" Miller — 20 years old, US Navy Corpsman 3rd class. Quick to smile, straight posture and no-nonsense. Nothing was more important to him than taking care of the wounded, their every need—and without hesitation. Did his job with precision and compassion. Respected by everyone.

Ski — 19 years old, US Marine Lance Corporal, Russian, Jewish kid, non-citizen, thick accent, single amputee and two front teeth knocked out from shrapnel. Easy going, but don't push him too far. Doesn't like to be the center of attention. Always optimistic, a peacemaker and longs to be a U.S. citizen.

Jeremy (Shoff) — 19 years old. US Navy sailor, injured in a car accident, guilt-ridden, ashamed of his choices for backing out of the Marines. Struggles to belong, wants to be accepted at all costs, but will stand his ground when challenged.

Earl Ray — 19 years old, US Marine lance corporal, and a triple amputee who never smiled, but constantly blew air up from the corner of his mouth. Handsome, with thick blond hair and a great cleft in his chin. Angry, always on the alert, proud, strong headed, in control of situations, but internally, he questions whether his life is worth living.

Dr. Donnolly	45, US Navy Commander, orthopedic surgeon, teacher and counselor and his only purpose was that of a surgeon. A casual, soft-spoken and dedicated compassionate healer.
Miss Berry	35 to 40 years old, US Navy Lt. Commander, Head nurse on Ward 2B. Five-feet six inches with a firm, full figure. Her jet-black hair bounced from the ever-present quickness in her steps. A constant smile that gave her a youthful look. Her love for nursing and caring for the wounded was more important than being a Navy officer. Motherly instincts.
Bobby Mac	22 years old, US Marine Sergeant, the oldest patient on the ward, combat-hardened, half-breed Cherokee. His ever-present jolliness at everything exuded his totally give-a-shit attitude. He brought a much-needed optimism and "bright-side" to any situation on the ward. His two years in combat had resulted in an unabashed, live-for-today exuberance.
Moose	19 years old, US. Marine corporal, double amputee, with a jovial, Hoss Cartwright-like stature and a broad, easy smile. He couldn't care less what other people thought of him, but he cared deeply for his fellow wounded Marines.
Ski's Poppa	50 years old. A small, thin, shy-looking Russian man with an extremely mild manner. A soft face and gold rim glasses that set tight on his narrow nose. He was constantly rolling his hat in his hands.

Roger	18 years old, US Marine lance corporal, injured in a motorcycle accident. Quiet and reserved and very giving.
Admiral	Late 50's. US Navy Admiral with a pompous attitude.
Big Al	20 years old, US Marine lance corporal with both legs completely gone up to his hips. Italian, with jet black hair, olive skin and a smile that never took a break, and anyone who came within talking distance was a friend.
Pappy	27 years old. US Coast Guard, 3rd class. He's been active duty for 7 years. Young-looking for his age. Quiet and a bit shy, and careful with his words. A below-the surface sadness for the wounded—but would never show it.
Bar Patron	40 something male with a hard-life look, a blue-collar frequent visitor to the Rainbow. Compassionate with a deep respect for the wounded.
Eva	30 years old. Bar owner of the Rainbow Bar and Grille with maturity beyond her years. Beautiful, slender with a feminine touch, but strong and independent. She had a love for all the wounded and a special tenderness for Earl Ray.
Rosie	30 years old. Owner of a high-end brothel, "Rosie's Place". Sure, confident and poised with a warm, calming and naturally seductive and flirtatious manner. She held a special place in her heart for all veterans and military. And a special place in her "home" for Big Al, Earl Ray and Jeremy.

Tiny	30 years old. US Navy Corpsman, First class. About 6'2" tall and 200 lbs. Easy-going, with a Captain Kangaroo look and mannerisms. Wounded in Vietnam, could have left the Navy, but re-enlisted to help the wounded. He had a deep compassion for those suffering and those he felt he had personally failed who had died under his care. A Santa Clause twinkle in his eyes.
Hippie	20 years old. Female with a hateful attitude toward the war and those in the military.
Sgt. Pepper	22 years old. US Marine sergeant and former patient at the Naval hospital. He turned against the war, the government and the military. Now a war protestor.
Dave	Mid-40's. Italian male, handsome, confident, a little brash and exuded authority. He radiated with the look of "money" and proved his respect with his generosity by providing entertainment for the wounded veterans.
Escort	Call girl. Early 20s. Classy, beautiful. The best Atlantic City had to offer.

CONTENTS

PRODUCTION NOTES...1

CASTING FOR NINE ACTORS / READERS THEATER SEATING CHART...3

PROPS
Suggested Backdrop Images...4, 5
Suggested Costumes...5
Prop List Suggestions by Scene:
Act I...6
Act II...7

SET DESIGN

ACT I
Act I, Scene 1: Incoming, 2B...8
Act I, Scene 2: Jennifer...8
Act I, Scene 3: The Fight...8
Act I, Scene 4: Ski's Big Day...8
Act I, Scene 5: The Club...8
Act I, Scene 6: The Admiral...8
Act I, Scene 7: The Solarium...8
Act I, Scene 8: Moving On...8

ACT II
Act II, Scene I: Q Ward...9
Act II, Scene 2: The Rainbow Bar & Grill...10
Act II, Scene 3: Getting Lucky...11
Act II, Scene 4: Rosie's Place...11
Act II, Scene 5: Back to Q...11
Act II, Scene 6: The Bus Ride...11
Act II, Scene 7: Atlantic City...10
Act II, Scene 8: Going Home...9
Act II, Scene 9: Shipping Out...10
Act II, Scene 10: Salute...9

COMPLETE SET AND PROP WISH LIST...12

THE STAGE PLAY 13

ACT I

Act I, Scene 1: Incoming, 2B...15
Act I, Scene 2: Jennifer...22
Act I, Scene 3: The Fight...30
Act I, Scene 4: Ski's Big Day...36
Act I, Scene 5: The Club...43
Act I, Scene 6: The Admiral...48
Act I, Scene 7: The Solarium...55
Act I, Scene 8: Moving On...62

ACT II

Act II, Scene I: Q Ward...65
Act II, Scene 2: The Rainbow Bar & Grill...75
Act II, Scene 3: Getting Lucky...82
Act II, Scene 4: Rosie's Place...91
Act II, Scene 5: Back to Q...95
Act II, Scene 6: The Bus Ride...99
Act II, Scene 7: Atlantic City...105
Act II, Scene 8: Going Home...111
Act II, Scene 9: Shipping Out...115
Act II, Scene 10: Salute...122

THE READERS THEATER VERSION 127

ACT I

Act I, Scene 1: Incoming, 2B...129
Act I, Scene 2: Jennifer...136
Act I, Scene 3: The Fight...144
Act I, Scene 4: Ski's Big Day...150
Act I, Scene 5: The Club...157
Act I, Scene 6: The Admiral...162
Act I, Scene 7: The Solarium...168
Act I, Scene 8: Moving On...175

ACT II

Act II, Scene I: Q Ward...178
Act II, Scene 2: The Rainbow Bar & Grill...188
Act II, Scene 3: Getting Lucky...194
Act II, Scene 4: Rosie's Place...203
Act II, Scene 5: Back to Q...207
Act II, Scene 6: The Bus Ride...211
Act II, Scene 7: Atlantic City...216
Act II, Scene 8: Going Home...222
Act II, Scene 9: Shipping Out...226
Act II, Scene 10: Salute...233

PRODUCTION NOTES

It is the author's dearest hope that groups of friends, college classes, community theater groups — anyone and everyone you can think of — will read this play aloud, to honor and remember not only the Marines who were his ward-mates during the two years they were patients together in the Philadelphia Naval Hospital, but *all* veterans who have served their country and came home profoundly affected by the things they saw, heard, did, and had done to them.

2025 is the 50th anniversary of the end of the war in Vietnam — the war in which the author's friends and fellow-patients served. This script can be used for free during that year only, on the condition that any funds collected would go to groups supporting disabled veterans, whether that group is Wounded Warriors or Operation Song or any other non-profit. For performances after 2025, please request permission and licensing from PurpleScribe68@gmail.com.

The play included in this book comes in two versions. The first half of the book includes a script for a fully mounted production, which can include any or all of the suggested props or stage direction suggestions. The second half is designed for readers theater — literally a group of readers lined up in chairs on a stage who read the words aloud from scripts that can be held or placed on stands in front of them, with a narrator reading the stage directions. There are lists of suggested props and the scenes in which they would be used, if any are used at all, and a chart for setting up those props. Another included chart shows a character breakdown which would allow either of these productions to make use of no more than nine actors plus a narrator, if one is needed.

The goal is for this remembrance to be as user-friendly as possible. Imagine the suggestions as a buffet. Take and use what you want… as long as you stay true to the words these soldiers spoke. Some of the countless possibilities are included on the next page. Use your imaginations. Just please read this book aloud and remember those who bravely served.

Some of the countless possibilities:

You could have nine readers plus a narrator lined up in a row of chairs, holding their scripts, never moving, just reading aloud.

You could have nine readers plus a narrator plus the images of the backdrops projected on a screen or wall behind them.

You could use the nine actors to do dramatic readings, rather than just reading the script aloud.

Your narrator could read the SETTING and AT RISE directions in addition to the ACTION directions, to help set the mood.

You could use parts of sets, or all or none of them.

You can turn Ward 2B into the solarium without moving anything, by doing nothing more than putting potted plants on the stools and ashtrays on the tables.

You can use folding chairs instead of wheelchairs and stools.

You can use your hands to mime talking on the phone instead of using rotary-dial phones.

You could do a fully-mounted production complete with sets, with stands by every chair so the readers could follow the scripts.

You could even do a fully-mounted production utilizing 21 actors in full costumes, in which the scripts are memorized and the scenes are acted out upon the stage.

A footlocker could be a coffee table, if you put a tablecloth over it. A costume change could be the actor playing BIG AL putting a coat and hat over his pajamas, to become SKI'S POPPA. EVA could become ROSIE by throwing on a robe and a boa.

You get the idea. You can do anything you can imagine.

Permission is granted for production of this play at any time in 2025, in any way you choose, as long as you remember these brave men and donate any proceeds to organizations supporting wounded veterans. After the end of 2025, please contact PurpleScribe68@gmail.com for production permission and licensing requirements. And always, always put on your play in memory of those who have served.

CASTING CHART FOR NINE ACTORS, BY SCENE

FOR READERS THEATER, ACTORS SIT IN THE FOLLOWING ORDER from stage left to stage right.
Add one chair off to either side of the stage for the NARRATOR.
If six wheelchairs are available, use for ACTORS/seats 1-3 and 7-9; use chairs or stools for 4-6.

	Act 1								Act 2									
Scene	1	2	3	4	5	6	7	8	1	2	3	4	5	6	7	8	9	10
	Incoming, 2B	Jennifer	The Fight	Ski's Big Day	The Club	The Admiral	The Solarium	Moving On	Q Ward	Rainbow B & G	Getting Lucky	Rosie's Place	Back to Q	The Bus Ride	Atlantic City	Going Home	Shipping Out	Salute
Actor(seat)/role																		
1. Moose			X	X	X	X	X	X	X	X				X	X	X	X	X
2. Big Al						X			X	X	X	X	X	X	X	X	X	X
Ski's Poppa				X														
Roger					X			X										
3. Earl Ray	X	X	X	X	X	X	X	X	X	X			X	X	X	X		
4. Dr Donnolly	X	X		X	X			X								X		
Admiral						X												
Pappy									X	X								X
Tiny														X	X			
5. Miss Barry	X	X		X	X	X		X										
Eva										X							X	
Rosie											X	X	X					
Hippie																X		
Escort															X			
6. Doc Miller	X	X	X	X	X	X		X										
Bar Patron										X							X	
Sgt Pepper															X			
Dave																X		
7. Ski	X	X	X	X	X	X	X	X	X	X				X	X	X	X	X
8. Jeremy	X	X	X	X	X	X	X	X	X	X	X	X	X	X	X	X	X	X
9. Bobby Mac		X	X	X	X	X	X	X	X	X				X	X	X	X	X

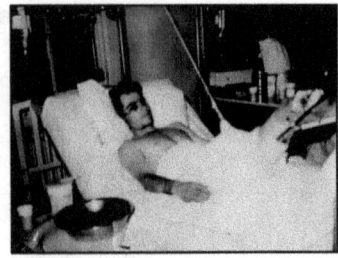

Act I, Scene 1:
Jeremy, Incoming, 2B

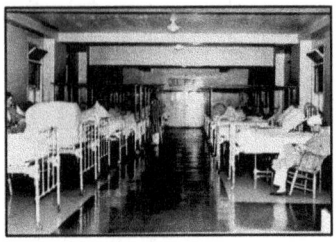

Act I, Scenes 2,3,4,5,6,8
Ward 2B

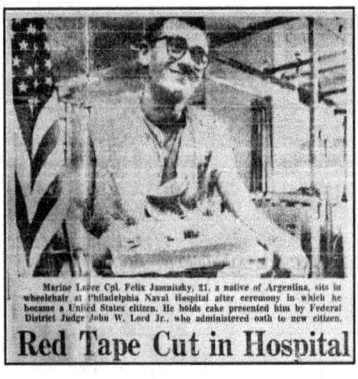

Act I, Scene 4 Citizenship

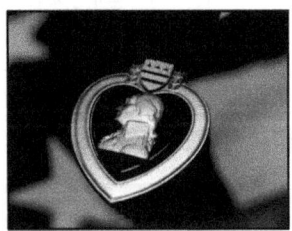

Act I, Scene 4: Purple Heart

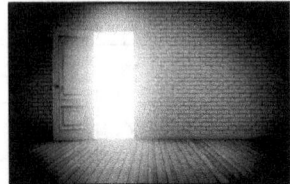

Act I, Scene 7: Solarium

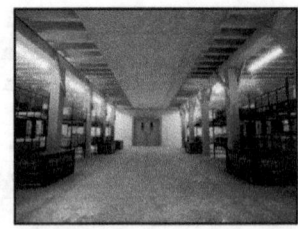

Act II, Scenes 1,8,10: Q Ward

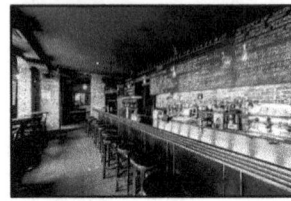

Act II, Scenes 2,9; Rainbow B&G

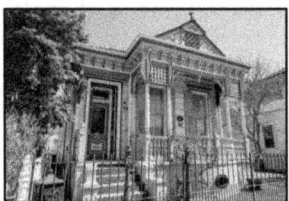

Act II, Scenes 3.4.5: Rosie's Place

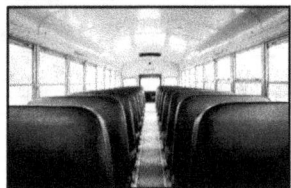

Act II, Scene 6: The Bus

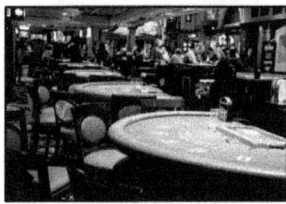

Act II, Scene 7: Atlantic City

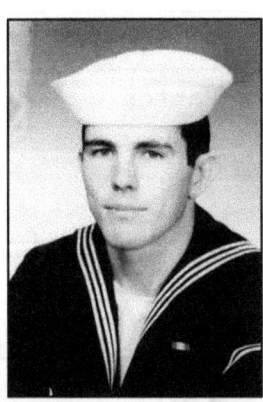

Act II, Scene 10: Jeremy, Salute

SUGGESTED BACKDROP IMAGES

Contact PurpleScribe68@gmail.com
for information about how to download the images.

Photo of Jeremy on Ward 2B: Act I Scene 1
Photo of Ward 2B interior: Act I Scenes 2,3,4,5,6,8
Photo of a flag: Act I Scene 4
Photo of a Purple Heart medal: Act I Scene 4
Photo of a glass wall of windows: Act I Scene 7
Photo of Q Ward: Act II Scenes 1,8
Photo of bar interior: Act II Scenes 2,9
Photo of the interior of Rosie's Place: Act II Scenes 3,4,5
Photo of a Navy bus: Act II Scene 6
Photo of classy lounge bar interior: Act II Scene 7
Photo of Jeremy in uniform: Act II Scene 10

SUGGESTED COSTUMES

Six sets of blue/white striped pajamas (JEREMY, SKI, EARL RAY, MOOSE, BOBBY MAC, and BIG AL for the entirety of Act I.)
Seven medical ID bracelets (for all patients, both Acts)
Five USMC non-dress khaki uniforms (MARINES, Act II.)
Three US Navy everyday white uniforms (DOC MILLER and MISS BERRY, Act I., and JEREMY, Act II.)
One US Navy Chief Petty Officer uniform (TINY)
One officer's uniform of US Navy everyday khakis (DONNOLLY)
One uniform for a US Navy admiral (the ADMIRAL)
One Coast Guard everyday uniform (PAPPY)
One set of white pajamas (ROGER)
Two pair white pajama pants (JEREMY and SKI, Act I.)
Two white balaclavas to serve as bandages for heads (JEREMY and ROGER, Act I.)
Six black cloth tubes closed at one end to cover amputated limbs: three legs below the knee, one leg above the knee, and two legs all the way up to the crotch
Two black cloth tubes closed at one end to cover one sleeve above the elbow and one below the elbow
Three white cloth tubes to cover two legs below the knees and one arm below the elbow
One large white bandage to cover the left eye (BOBBY MAC)
One set of Marine fatigues covered by fringed vest and peace emblems) and one 60s female hippie (SGT PEPPER and HIPPIE)
One female brothel owner (ROSIE)
One female bar owner (EVA)
One rich, well dressed Mafia member (DAVE)
One call girl (ESCORT)
One coat and cap (SKI's POPPA)
One regular 1960s guy in a bar (BAR PATRON)

SUGGESTED PROP LIST BY SCENE.

All scenes would benefit from a white screen backdrop and a way to project the backdrop images onto the screen with or without the use of any additional props.

ACT I

Scene 1: Incoming, 2B
- Photo of patient on Ward 2B
- Six wheelchairs
- Three stools
- Two small tables
- One battery-operated drill
- Nine stands

Scene 2: Jennifer
- Photo of Ward 2B
- Six wheelchairs
- Three stools
- Two small tables
- One rotary dial phone
- Nine stands

Scene 3: The Fight
- Photo of Ward 2B
- Six wheelchairs
- Three stools
- Two small tables
- One folder
- One rotary dial phone
- Nine stands

Scene 4: Ski's Big Day
- Photo of Ward 2B
- One comb
- Photo of a flag
- Photo of a Purple Heart medal
- Five wheelchairs
- One chair
- Three stools
- Two small tables
- One small gift-wrapped box
- One framed certificate
- Nine stands

Scene 5: The Club
- Photo of Ward 2B
- Six wheelchairs
- Three stools
- Two small tables
- Nine stands
- One pair of crutches

Scene 6: The Admiral
- Photo of Ward 2B
- Six wheelchairs
- Three stools
- Two small tables
- One rotary dial telephone
- Nine stands

Scene 7: The Solarium
- Photo of a glass wall of windows
- Six wheelchairs
- Three stools
- Two small tables
- Two to five potted plants
- Two ashtrays
- Six stands
- One Jack Daniels bottle
- Six hand-rolled cigarettes
- A packet
- A crumpled letter
- A few Polaroid photos

Scene 8: Moving On
- Photo of Ward 2B
- Six wheelchairs
- Three stools
- Two small tables
- Nine stands

ACT II

Scene 1: Q Ward
Photo of Q Ward
Full-length mirror on a stand
Six wheelchairs
One stool
One footlocker
Assorted prosthetic arms/legs
One Navy sea bag
One Coast Guard duffel bag

Scene 2: Rainbow Bar & Grille
Photo of bar interior
Three bar-height tables
Nine stools
Three stands
Seven beer pitchers
Seven mugs
One tray

Scene 3: Getting Lucky
Photo of hanging bead curtain
Two wheelchairs
Two purple chairs
One purple couch
One coffee table
One lamp with fringed shade
One ashtray
Pack of cigarettes
Lighter
Two mugs of beer
Three glasses of wine
Five stands

Scene 4: Rosie's Place
Photo of hanging bead curtain
Two wheelchairs
One small table
Two large padded chairs
One padded couch
One coffee table
One ashtray
One lamp with fringed shade
Two rotary-dial phone
Five stands

Scene 5: Back to Q
Photo of hanging bead curtain
Two purple chairs
One purple couch
One coffee table
One lamp with fringed shade
One ashtray
One pair of crutches
Two prosthetic legs and one arm

Scene 6: The Bus Ride
Photo of a Navy bus
Seven wheelchairs
Seven stands
One prosthetic arm with hook

Scene 7: Atlantic City
Photo of a classy hotel lounge
Six chairs
Two wheelchairs
Two prosthetic legs and one arm
Three card-table sized tables
Assorted bottles of liquor/mixers
Three trays
Seven fancy liquor glasses

Scene 8: Going Home
Photo of Q Ward
Six wheelchairs
One stool
One footlocker
One bottle of Jack Daniels
Two prosthetic legs and one arm
One small box
One pill bottle
One bundle of letters
One rotary-dial phone
Six stands

Scene 9: Shipping Out
Photo of lounge bar interior
Three small tables
Six chairs
Several trays, mugs, and
    pitchers of beer

Scene 10: Salute
Photo of Jeremy in uniform
Six wheelchairs
Two prosthetic legs and one arm
One stool
One footlocker
One sea bag
One crumpled letter
Six stands

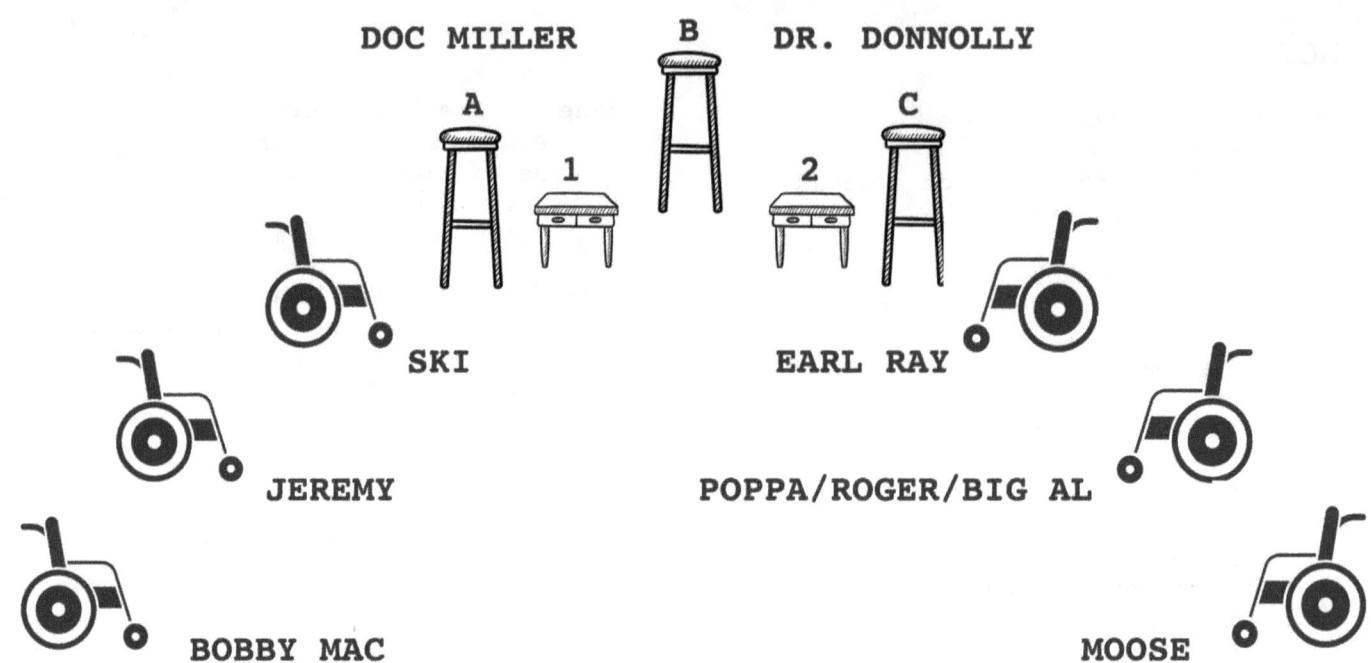

ACT I, ALL SCENES

Scene 1: Battery Operated Drill on Table 2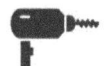

Scene 2: Rotary-dial Phone on Table 1

Scene 3: Rotary-dial Phone, Folder/Chart on Table 1

Scene 4: Comb on Table 1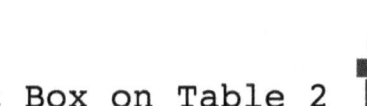

Certificate and Gift Box on Table 2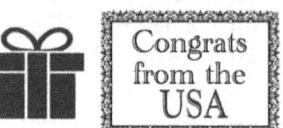

Small Box in Earl Ray's Pocket

Scene 5: No additional props

Scene 6: Rotary-dial Phone on Table 1

Scene 7: Potted plants on Tables 1 and 2 and Stools A, B, C

Scene 8: No additional props

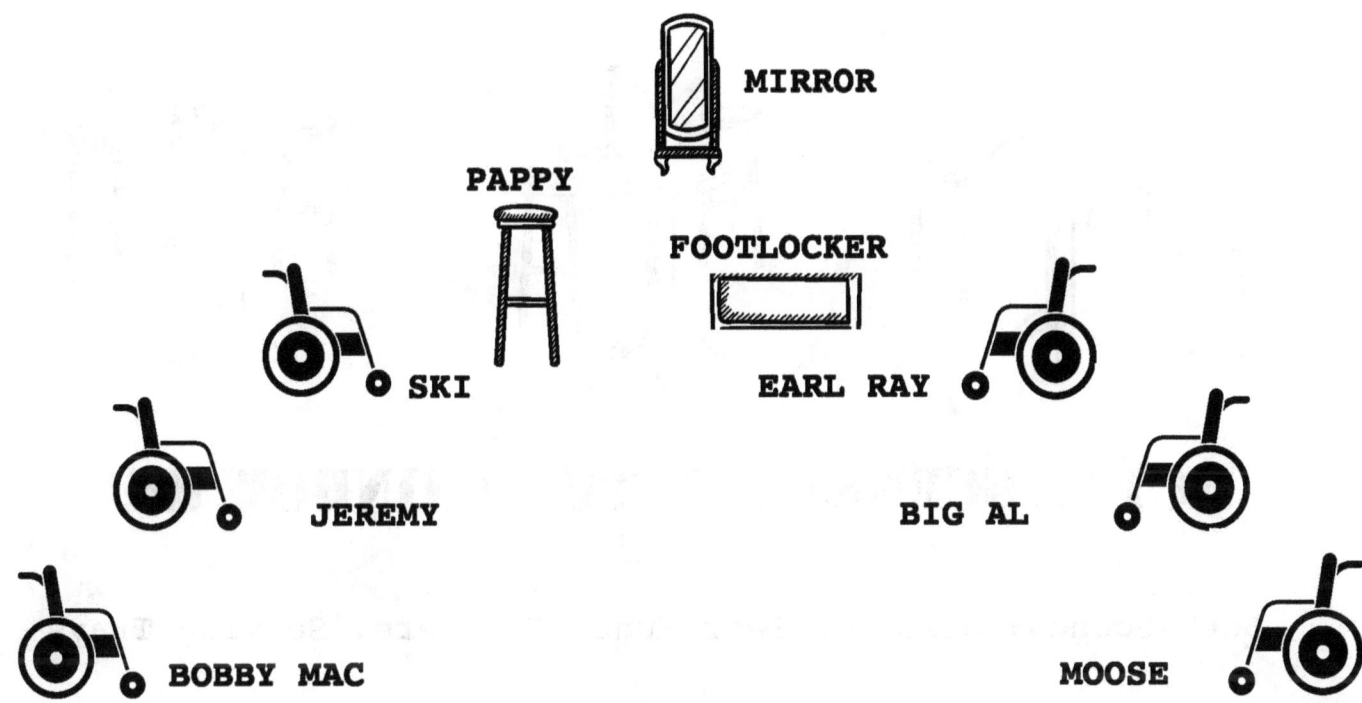

ACT II, SCENES 1, 8, 10: WARD Q

Scene 1: PAPPY carries Duffle Bag

BOBBY MAC carries Hand

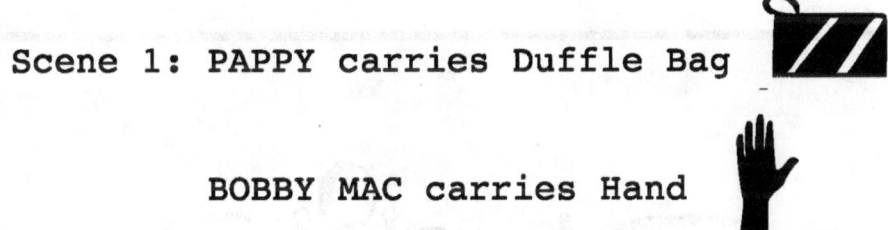

Scene 8: Bundle of Letters, Pill Bottle, Jack Daniels Bottle, and Small Box on Footlocker

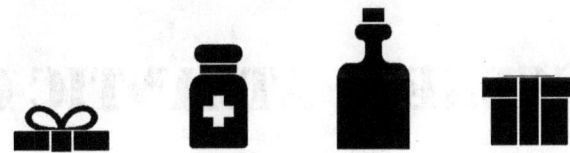

Scene 10: JEREMY carries Duffle Bag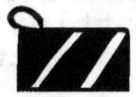

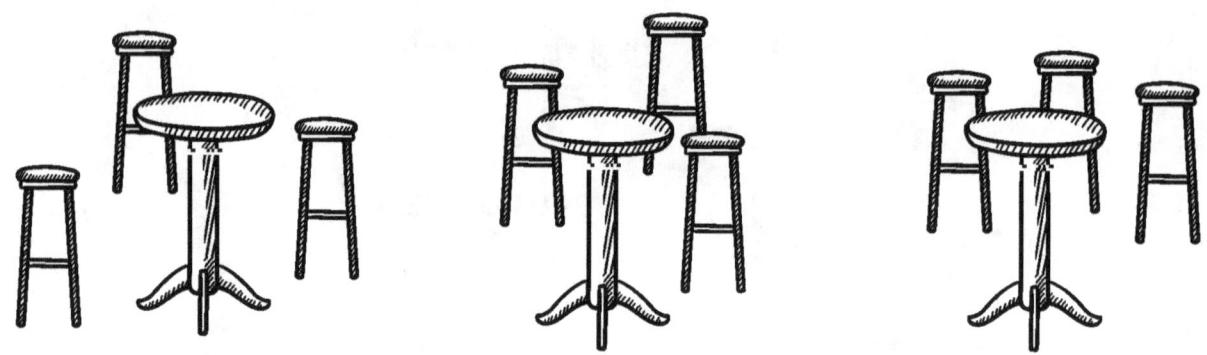

ACT II, SCENES 2, 9: THE RAINBOW B&G

Both Scenes: Assorted Beer Mugs, Pitchers, Serving Trays

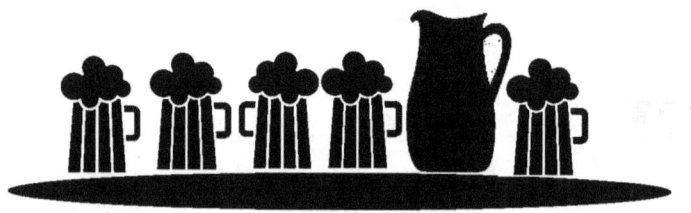

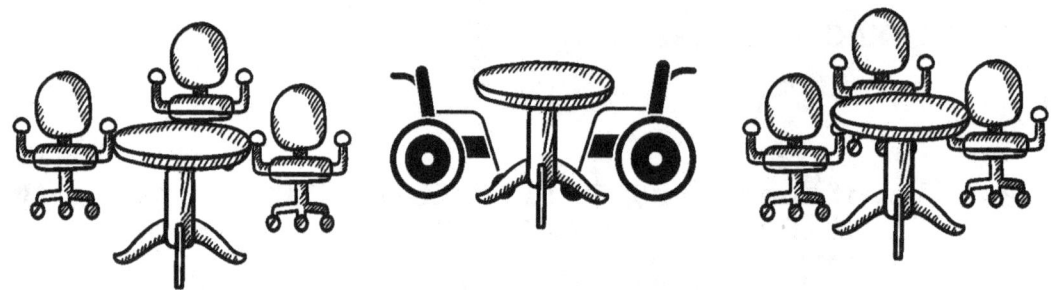

ACT II, SCENE 7: ATLANTIC CITY

Assorted Trays,
Liquor Bottles, Glasses,
Cigarettes

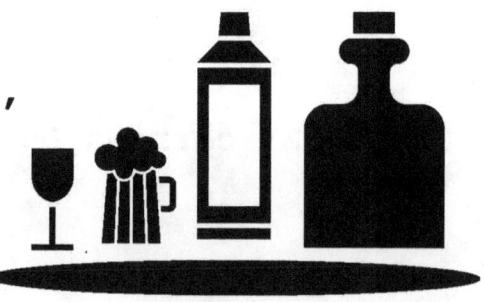

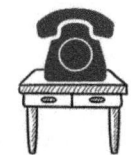
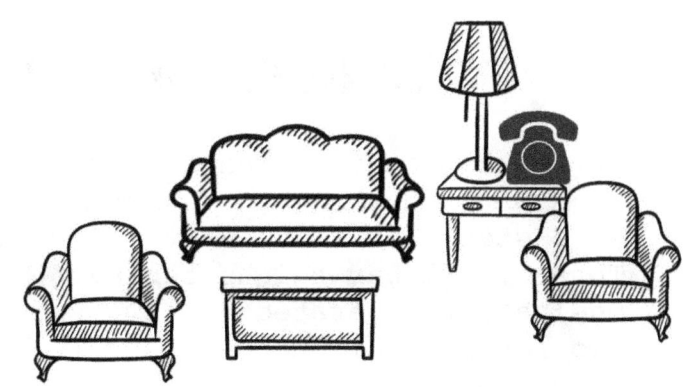
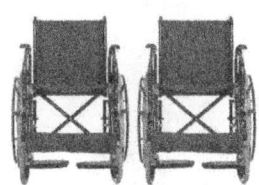

ACT II, SCENES 3, 4, 5: ROSIE'S PLACE

Scene 3: Cigarette Pack, Lighter, Tray, Two Beer Mugs, Three Wine Glasses

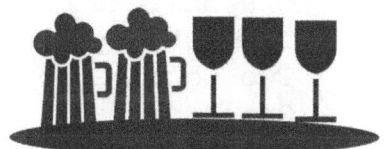

Scene 5: One Pair of Crutches

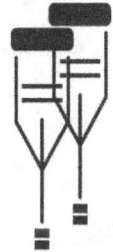

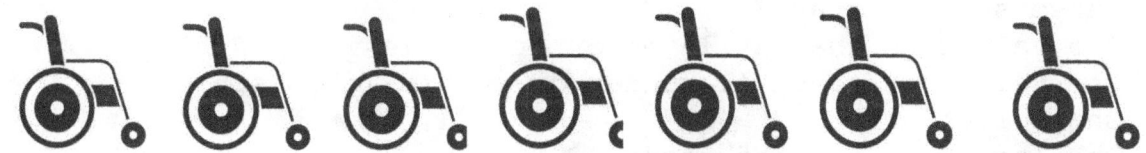

JEREMY, SKI, BOBBY MAC, MOOSE, BIG AL, EARL RAY, TINY

ACT II, SCENE 6: THE BUS

Scene 6: No additional Props

COMPLETE SET AND PROP WISH LIST

Seven wheelchairs (Can be borrowed or rented from medical supply stores. In Nashville, one rental is about $50/week.)
Nine stools
Three small bar-height tables
One battery-operated drill
Two rotary-dial phones
Nine stands for scripts
Six chairs
Two small boxes, one with a bow on it
One framed certificate
One comb
One pair of crutches
Two ashtrays
Two to five potted plants, live or plastic
One Jack Daniels bottle
Several hand-rolled cigarettes
One large envelope
One slightly crumpled letter/envelope
A few Polaroid photos
One full-length mirror on a stand
One footlocker
One Navy sea bag
One Coast Guard duffel bag
Three tables, card table sized
Assorted bottles of liquor and mixers
Seven fancy liquor glasses
Several beer pitchers
Seven beer mugs
Three wine glasses
Three serving trays
Two velveteen chairs (lavender or purple if possible)
One velveteen couch (lavender or purple if possible)
One coffee table
One lamp with fringed shade
One pack of cigarettes
One cigarette lighter
One prescription pill bottle
One bundle of letters
One crumpled sheet of paper
One white free-standing screen with a stand and projector
IF POSSIBLE: One rubber hand, at least two prosthetic legs, and one prosthetic arm with hook. Request loans from your local AMVETs or VFW. The total number of prosthetic arms and legs used by the patients on the ward is three arms and six legs.

PURPLE HEARTS

based on the novel
How Can You Mend This Purple Heart
by
Terry L. Gould

stage play adaptation by
Terry L. Gould and M.C. Nelson

To contact Terry Gould,
email:
purplescribe68@gmail.com

Cast Of Characters

Doc Miller:	Navy hospital corpsman. Age 20.
Ski:	Russian-born patient. USMC. Age 19.
Jeremy:	Patient. Navy. Age 19.
Earl Ray:	Patient. USMC. Age 19.
Dr. Donnolly:	Navy orthopedic surgeon. Mid 40s.
Miss Berry:	Navy Lt. Commander. Late 30s.
Bobby Mac:	Patient. USMC. Pt Cherokee. Age 22.
Moose:	Patient. USMC. Age 19.
Ski's Poppa:	Immigrant. Russian. Mid 50s.
Roger:	Patient. USMC. Age 19.
Admiral:	Officer with an attitude.
Big Al:	Patient. USMC. Age 20.
Pappy:	Patient. US Coast Guard. Age 27.
Bar Patron:	Any age bar patron.
Eva:	Bar owner. Early 30s.
Rosie:	Brothel owner. Early 30s.
Tiny:	Navy Chief Petty Officer. Mid-30s.
Hippie:	Female war protester. Early 20s.
Sgt. Pepper:	USMC war protester. Early 20s.
Dave:	Mafioso. Mid-40s.
Escort:	Call girl. Early 20s.
Off-screen Voices:	Can be read by any offstage actor.

Scene

U.S. Naval Hospital and other sites in Philadelphia, Pennsylvania, and Atlantic City, New Jersey.

Time

1969, early in the Vietnam War.

ACT I

SCENE 1

SETTING: *Ward 2B. A photo of a patient on a naval hospital ward is projected onto a screen behind the actors.*

In an arc across the stage from stage right to stage left are: an empty wheelchair, JEREMY dozing in a wheelchair, a space for SKI's wheelchair, a stool for DOC MILLER, a small table, a stool where MISS BERRY is sitting, a small table with a battery operated drill, DR. DONNOLLY sitting on a stool, EARL RAY in a wheelchair, and two more empty wheelchairs. In front of each seat is a stand for the script.

AT RISE: *The lights come up on each seat in order from stage right to stage left. DOC MILLER comes in pushing SKI in his wheelchair to the empty spot, then sits on the empty stool.*

DOC MILLER
Okay, Ski, Dr. Donnolly'll be in to see you in a little while. He's the one who put your legs back together. In the meantime, we'll get you another needle to help you relax.

SKI gives a thumbs up.

JEREMY (*waking*)
What's happening? Who are these people? Dear God, what is this place? Am I in Hell?

DOC MILLER
Easy, Shoff. You're not in Hell. Well, not exactly. You're in the Philly Naval Hospital. You're here 'cause you were in a car wreck three days ago and almost died. You needed the best orthopedist we've got, so they brought you here. You're in good hands with Dr. Donnolly. He treats the Marines back from Nam.

JEREMY
These guys here. That's who they are, aren't they? They're Marines who were wounded in Vietnam, aren't they? <u>Aren't they</u>! I should have been in Vietnam with them instead of joining the Navy. I should never have backed out of joining the Marines. I should have been one of them. I am so ashamed that I wasn't. That I took the easy way out. I don't deserve to be in the same room with them. To be in their presence. Oh, God, I am so ashamed.

I-1-2

> *EARL RAY looks over and
> gives JEREMY the finger.*

       EARL RAY
Noncombat motherfucker.

       SKI
Felix Dawntay dJamnitzky.

       JEREMY
What?

       SKI
Felix Dawntay dJamnitzky. Allld my friends call me Skee.

       JEREMY
Jeremy Shoff. All my friends just call me Shoff.

       SKI
dYou look like sheet.

       JEREMY
What?

       SKI
dYou look like sheet.

       JEREMY
You don't look much better. What happened to land you in here?
      (*pause*)
Maybe I shouldn't have --

       SKI
Eet's okay. Eet's just that my leg, eet burns sometimes. Eet was a land mine. My buddy tripped dthe wire. He took most of dthe blast. Died instdantly.

       JEREMY
Where're you from?

       SKI
dNew Jersey.

       JEREMY
No, really. Where're you from?

       SKI
I was born in dRussia. Someday, I want to be ceetizen here.

       DOC MILLER
Okay, Ski, here's that morphine for you. Let's see that bulldog tattoo. You choose. Where should that bulldog get it this time? How about right between the eyes?

SKI
I don't care. Just geeve eet to me.

DOC MILLER
How about you, Shoff? You need anything? If you do, just ask for me. The name's Randy Miller, but you know us corpsmen; we like to think we're more than glorified medics. Everyone here just calls me Doc.

JEREMY
Yeah, Doc. As soon as you can.

DOC MILLER
You've got it. I'll be back in a little while to bring it and check on you two. Oh! I almost forgot. You had a buddy who came to see you before he shipped out. I think his name was Bill?

JEREMY
My best friend. He had more sense than to go out partying with us the night we graduated, so he was spared being in the wreck.

DOC MILLER
He said to tell you the two in the back seat were sent to Aberdeen. Two others are here, on a different ward, and are doing well. But the driver, well, he didn't make it. And your friend must know you well, because he said for you to not give us any trouble.

JEREMY (*laughing*)
Yeah. Like I would do that.

DOC MILLER
You need anything while I'm getting out the shots, Earl Ray?

EARL RAY
(*gives DOC the finger*)
What the hell do you think, Doc?

JEREMY
You really from Russia, Ski?

SKI
dYep.

JEREMY
What's Russia like?

SKI
I don't dknow. We moved here when I was leetle. My parents let me enlist. I am not a ceetizen yet. But someday, I hope.

DR. DONNOLLY
Hello, Ski. I'm Dr. Donnolly, and this is Lt. Commander Dorothy Berry.
(MORE)

                    DR. DONNOLLY (CONT'D)
Miss Berry is the head nurse for this floor and she's going to
help me take a look at you. I know this is going to hurt, but
you could have been paralyzed, Ski, and I need to see what we
have back there.
                    (*pause*)
It looks pretty good, considering. Unfortunately, we can't remove
that piece of shrapnel from the back of your throat. It's too
dangerous.

                    SKI
Eeet doesn't hurt that much, sir.

                    DR. DONNOLLY
That's good to know. Now I need to take a look inside your legs.
If it gets to be too much, we'll stop. Just let me know.

                    SKI
Eeets okay.

                    DR. DONNOLLY
The shrapnel shattered both of your shin bones, so we attached
steel rods to them, leaving gaps in the bones between your ankles
and knees. As your shin bones grow, we can compress the rods
from out here. That assists the fusion. Right now we need to
change the dressings on your legs. It's going to be uncomfortable.

                    MISS BERRY
Are you doing okay, Ski?

                    SKI
Yes, ma'am. Eets okay.

                    MISS BERRY
Let me know if this gets to be too much, Ski. We've got all day.

                    SKI (*writhing*)
Eet's okay, ma'am.

                    JEREMY
Take my hand, Ski!

          SKI grabs Jeremy's hand.

                    MISS BERRY
Hold on, Ski. We're almost finished. Just two more. Can we get
him something, Doctor?

                    DR. DONNOLLY
Bring me a half dose of morphine, Randy. We're going to need to
change that dressing three times a day, Ski, so if it gets to be
too much at any time, just let us know.

                                    SKI
Eets okay, sir.

                                    JEREMY
I can't believe how you handled that, Ski. I couldn't have done
it. Not one word from all that pain.

                                    SKI
Eeet wasn't that bad. Not as bad as that fawcking land mine.
Thanks for your hand. I hope I didn't squeeze too hard. I sure
could use a cigdarette.

                                    DOC MILLER
Sorry, Ski. You're not allowed to smoke right after a needle.
You might drop your cigarette and burn yourself.

                                    SKI
What in the hell dwe supposed to do?

                                    DOC MILLER (*laughing*)
Just ask for another needle. No tobacco after a shot, but
unlimited morphine. We give it out like candy. Just ask.

                                    DR. DONNOLLY
Randy, can you get me a sterile gown pack?

                                    DOC MILLER
Yes, sir. Is it time, sir?

                                    DR. DONNOLLY
Yes. Thanks, Randy. I think it's time. Is everyone ready?

                                    MISS BERRY/DOC
We're ready.

                                    SKI
Uh-oh, Shoff. It looks like dyou are dnext.

                                    DR. DONNOLLY
Jeremy, now that your concussion is clear, we need to get this
leg into traction. To do that, we have to pull your leg tight to
keep the broken ends of your femur from scraping together or
cutting into your thigh muscle. We'll insert this pin crossways
through your shin bone, just below your knee. It's going to be
uncomfortable, but it should only take a few minutes.

                                    JEREMY
Oh, shit. Sorry, sir.

                                    DR. DONNOLLY
It's okay. We're giving you a special pain medication that should
help, which should last just a little longer than it will take us
to finish.

*DR DONNOLLY carries the drill over
to stand in front of JEREMY, his
back to the audience, holding the
drill hidden between them. He then
turns it on for a few moments.*

JEREMY (*writhing*)

AAUGH!

*Sobbing, Jeremy covers
his face with his hands.*

DR. DONNOLLY

Breathe, Shoff! Breathe now!
         (*pause*)
Sorry, Jeremy, just a couple of mechanical adjustments, and we'll be done. I know it hurt. I wouldn't want to have to go through it myself.

MISS BERRY

We'll have something ready for your pain in just a few minutes. In the meantime, I think we need to remove some of the glass from that cut in your head. Let's get that bandage off you.

*DOC MILLER Removes JEREMY's
balaclava.*

JEREMY

How's it look, Doc?

DOC MILLER

Wow. Too bad these aren't diamonds. We could make a fortune.

JEREMY

I'm sorry I yelled like that, Ski. You set the bar too high.

SKI

I just dthink I'm used to it by now. Dyou should have heard me when the land mine exploded.

EARL RAY

He didn't hear anything, 'cause he's a noncombat motherfucker.

JEREMY

Okay. I've seen your hateful looks, and I've heard them call you Earl Ray, so let's get this over with, Earl. I'm Jeremy Shoff, radioman, US Navy. I'm here 'cause the night before I was supposed to ship out I got drunk and was in a car wreck.

SKI

Felix Dawntay dJamnitzky. Lance dCorporal, U.-S.-M.-C., first battalion, seventh dMarines. A bad land mine.

                    EARL RAY
Why don't you just give him your fucking serial number while you're
at it? Shit, you don't know what a fucking bad land mine is.
                    (*points at right leg stump*)
Bad land mine, my ass.

                    SKI
Just geeve eet a break, Earl.

                    EARL RAY
Hey, noncombat motherfucker, do you know what it's like to kill
somebody? I didn't think so. I can't believe I'm in here with a
noncombat sissy motherfucker. Of all the bullshit fucking things
to happen to me. You even smell like a noncombat motherfucker,
Shoff. Somebody get me some noncombat motherfuckin' air freshener.

                    SKI
Geeve eet a fauwcking break, Earl.

                    JEREMY
It's okay, Ski. Let it go. Maybe it makes him feel better.

                    EARL RAY
The only thing that would make me feel better is your noncombat
ass out of my sight.

                    JEREMY
Then have them move your ass over to another ward.

                    EARL RAY
Why you smart-ass motherfucker!

                    JEREMY
No more than you, Earl.

                    SKI
Okay, dyou two. Geeve eet a break. Why don't dyou two just keese
and make up?

                    EARL RAY
Noncombat motherfucker can kiss my ass.

            Lights fade and go out,
            one at a time, stage right
            to stage left.

ACT I

SCENE 2

SETTING: *A few weeks later on Ward 2B. A photo of the ward is projected onto the screen behind the actors.*

In an arc across the stage from stage right are: an empty space for BOBBY MAC; JEREMY and SKI in wheelchairs; a stool for DOC MILLER; a small table holding a rotary dial telephone and a folder; MISS BERRY on a stool; a small table; DR. DONNOLLY sitting on a stool; EARL RAY in a wheelchair; and two empty wheelchairs. In front of each seat is a stand for the script.

AT RISE: *As lights come up, one at a time, stage right to stage left, DOC MILLER pushes in BOBBY MAC in his wheelchair, parks him next to JEREMY, then sits on his stool.*

DOC MILLER
Let's see here.
    (*picks up and looks at folder*)
Not too bad for what could have happened. Says here you jumped on a live grenade to save your buddies. You could have lost your head.

BOBBY MAC
What makes you think I didn't?

DOC MILLER
'Cause I can still see it. Randy Miller. Everyone calls me 'Doc.'

BOBBY MAC
Bobby Mac Joyce. Nice to know you, Doc. I'd shake your hand, but you'd have to go to Nam to get it.

DOC MILLER
Well, you're in luck, Bobby Mac Joyce. You still have your thumb. The whole thing.

BOBBY MAC
Well, ain't that some shit. They told me on the chopper I lost my whole arm.
    (*to JEREMY*)
Hey, man. I can tell you ain't combat. What the fuck happened to you?

JEREMY
The name's Shoff. Car hit a bridge.

BOBBY MAC
That fucking car wreck kicked your ass.

JEREMY
Yeah. But it ain't shit compared to you guys.

BOBBY MAC
Yeah, well, ain't a fucking thing we can do about it now. They let you smoke in here?

DOC MILLER
Need to put 'em down, Bobby. I gotta get your vitals. Can't have the smoke messing up the numbers.

BOBBY MAC
Shit, Doc. Just fill in some numbers. I'm breathing, ain't I?

DOC MILLER
No can do, Bobby Mac. Give me your right arm so I can get your B-P. Need anything for pain?

BOBBY MAC
Better get a couple more of those shots ready, Doc, I'll need more soon. I used to have two or three before breakfast in Nam.

DOC MILLER
Brag all you want, but I can tell you're not a junkie. You're in great shape and that's probably what kept you from being any worse.

BOBBY MAC
Any worse? Shit, this is heaven! Got me a hotel room, a bed with clean sheets, and somebody bringing me drugs all day and night. Don't get any better than this, man.

DR. DONNOLLY
Let's take a look in that eye socket, Bobby. It's looking pretty good. How's it feel?

BOBBY MAC
Like there's a hole where there shouldn't be a hole. It's kind of drafty.

DR. DONNOLLY
It won't be too long before we can fit you with a replacement.

BOBBY MAC (*laughing*)
In the meantime, I'll keep an eye out for you.

DR. DONNOLLY
That was absolutely terrible, Bobby. How're you doing, Ski?

                              SKI
Eet's okay, sir.

                          DR. DONNOLLY
We need to get another set of x-rays and see how well we're doing.
I won't make another adjustment for a couple more days. Give you
a little break.

                              SKI
Thdank you, sir. Eet doesn't hurt all that bad.

                          DR. DONNOLLY
Thank you, young man.
          (to EARL RAY)
Your arm is starting to look a lot better, Earl. Soon, we'll be
able to start measuring for your new arm.

                           EARL RAY
Yeah. I can hardly wait.

                          DR. DONNOLLY
Let me have a look at the rest of you.

                           EARL RAY
You mean what's left of me.

                          DR. DONNOLLY
We're going to have you walking before you know it, Earl.

                           EARL RAY
Easy for you to say. I've been here too long already.

                          DR. DONNOLLY
The past six months must seem like forever, Earl, but you're doing
really well. You only need a couple more minor surgeries and
we'll be able to get you out onto the rehab wards.

                           EARL RAY
Oh, yeah? I'm doing well compared to <u>what</u>?

                          DR. DONNOLLY
Look, Earl, I can't imagine how you feel. But I --

                           EARL RAY
No, you can't! Ain't nobody can know how I feel! Jesus H. Christ!

                          DR. DONNOLLY
Earl, that's not going to help you. I need you to be positive
about this. <u>You</u> need it, too.

                           EARL RAY
Gimme that needle, Doc. I need to escape this shit.

                              DOC MILLER
Here you go, Earl.

                              EARL RAY
That all you got?

                              DOC MILLER
That's it, Earl. I can't wait for this to put you out.

                              EARL RAY
Me, neither. Hey, noncombat motherfucker, what do you do in the
Navy, scrub floors? Kiss my ass, noncombat motherfucker.

                              JEREMY
You kiss my ass, Earl. What do you want me to do, have 'em cut
my legs off? You've got a lot of reasons to hate me, Earl. It's
okay. I don't blame you. I'd hate me, too, if I were you. Or
maybe I wouldn't. A lot of these guys in here are looking at
life in a wheelchair, and they don't hate me. It's just you,
Earl. You're the one full of hate, and you're always directing
it at me.

                              EARL RAY
Fuck you, Shoff. Can't wait to get my ass out of here. Me and
my girlfriend Jen, we'll pick up where we left off.

                              SKI
Dyou are verdy lucky guy. My girlfriend told me to djust be
careful, and I never heard from her again.

                              EARL RAY
What was her name?

                              SKI
I don't dremember. My first time to get laid was in Nam.

                              EARL RAY
I never touched the stuff. Jen's the only one for me.

                              SKI
That's why dyou are very lucky.

                              EARL RAY
Yeah. We'll see how lucky I am. Hey, Shoff, you got a girl?

                              JEREMY
Not any more. And thanks for not calling me a noncombat
motherfucker.

                              EARL RAY
Don't be so happy, Shoff. You'll always be a noncombat
motherfucker to me. What'd she do, Shoff? Your girl?

                              JEREMY
She sent me a "Dear John" while I was in boot camp. Said we didn't
have a lot in common anymore. I found out later she was screwing
a guy at college who was getting an education and had a Corvette.
I just keep trying to figure out why I wasn't good enough.

                               SKI
Sounds dlike you were pretty serious. How long deed you go with
her?

                              JEREMY
Just over a year. I thought we were headed for the altar. She's
the one who talked me out of joining the Marines with my best
friend.

                             EARL RAY
That's life, man. Look at you now. A noncombat motherfucker
laid up in here with me just twelve feet away. You join the Navy
to see the world and what you get is a world of shit. And that
girlfriend fucked you twice.

                              JEREMY
Say what?

                             EARL RAY
Your girl. She fucked you twice. She left you for some school
boy on campus <u>and</u> she talked you out of being with your buddy in
the Corps.

                              JEREMY
Yeah, Earl. That was my mistake.

            MISS BERRY picks up phone.

                            MISS BERRY
                    (*into phone*)
2B.
                    (*pause*)
Yes. He's here.
                    (*pause*)
I understand. All I can do is ask.
                    (*pause*)
Yes, hold on.
                         (*MISS BERRY carries the
                          phone to EARL RAY. Holds
                          the handset out to him as
                          she continues to hold the
                          base.*)
It's for you, Earl. It's Jennifer again. She's at the gate.
Again. Please talk to her, Earl. Just talk to her. Just give
her a chance. She's been writing and calling you and coming here
for almost a year. She's proved to you that she hasn't given up
on you and isn't likely to. Please, give her a chance. Please.

> *EARL RAY accepts the handset. MISS BERRY holds the base as he looks at her, looks at the handset, and finally answers.*

EARL RAY
Hello, Jen. It's me. Earl.
> (*pause*)

I love you, too, Jen, but you love another Earl. The old Earl. I'm not the same person you knew before.
> (*pause*)

You don't understand. I know you've been talking with my mother and you think you know how bad it is, but whatever it is you're imagining, it's worse.
> (*pause*)

You think the two of you have it worked out? You really think you're ready? Because I'm <u>not</u> ready, Jen. I'm just not.
> (*pause*)

You're the <u>only</u> thing keeping me sane, Jen, but I'm still not ready. Did you ever think of that?
> (*pause*)

Okay, Jen. I give up. You can come in. Just ask for Miss Berry when you get to the desk and give me a few minutes. I'll come.

> *Earl hands the handset back to Miss Berry, who puts phone back on table.*

MISS BERRY
It'll be okay, Earl. I'll go take care of everything.

> *Miss Berry exits behind screen.*

SKI
Anything you want to talk about, before Jendifer gets up here?

EARL RAY
I don't think I'm ready, Ski. What is she going to think when she sees a guy with one arm and no legs?

SKI
Eet'll be okay, Earl. She loves dyou and dyou are very lucky.

EARL RAY
Jesus. Why did I agree to this? I'm not who she thinks I am.

SKI
A dMarine is aldways ready, my friend. Eet will be fine. Dwe are all with you.

EARL RAY
Thanks, Ski.

I-2-14

MISS BERRY returns to the stage and sits on her stool.

MISS BERRY
Okay, Earl. Jennifer is the Solarium, whenever you're ready to join her there. Is there anything else I can do to help?

EARL RAY
No, ma'am. I can do this. All I have to do is get myself in there, let go of the chair, put my arm around her, and tell her that I love her. I can do this. Let go of the chair. Put my arm around her. Tell her --

DOC MILLER
You want me to give you a push, Earl?

EARL RAY
No. I have to do this myself. I have to.

EARL RAY propels his wheelchair towards the screen using his one hand, talking to himself as he goes.

EARL RAY
Get myself in there. Let go of the chair. Put my arm around her. Tell her that I love her.

As EARL RAY goes behind the screen, there is a loud crash and a thud.

EARL RAY (*shouting*)
Jen! Jen! Miss Berry! Doc! Come quick! Please! Help! Help!

MISS BERRY and DOC rush behind the screen. DOC runs back out and grabs an empty wheelchair, pushing it behind the screen. MISS BERRY slowly pushes EARL RAY back to his place.

EARL RAY
Oh, Miss Berry. Jen. Jen. Is she going to be okay?

MISS BERRY
I think she'll be fine, Earl, but she's going to need a few stitches where she hit her head on the table as she fainted. Randy will take her down to the emergency room, and will let us know what the doctor says.

EARL RAY
I should never have let her see me. It's all my fault.

MISS BERRY
She was just surprised, Earl. That's all. She was just surprised.
She'll be okay. Just give her some time.

EARL RAY
I should never have let her see what is left of me. I shouldn't
have told her she could come up. I knew neither of us was ready.

SKI
Eeet will be okay when she comes back up, Earl. You two weel be
fine.

EARL RAY
I don't think I can make it without her, Ski.

*DOC MILLER comes back on
the ward, pushing the empty
wheelchair to its place.*

DOC MILLER
She's doing fine, Earl. The doctor on duty wants her under
observation for a couple of hours, and then he's going to send
her back to the motel to rest. There was no serious injury, they
just want to make sure. Her mother is going to come pick her up.
She will call you as soon as she feels better. She promised.

*EARL RAY starts hitting
his one good arm on the
arm of his chair.*

EARL RAY
No she won't! I know she won't! Fuck 'em. Fuck all of 'em. I
don't give a shit about any of 'em. I didn't need her letters in
Nam and I sure as hell don't need her help now. She and her mother
can kiss my ass! All of you can kiss my ass!

SKI
Did Dmarines help dyou in Nam, Earl?

EARL RAY
That's a stupid fucking question. Of course they did. We helped
each other right up until some asshole medics thought it was a
good idea to save my worthless life. That didn't help at all.
Now. You got any more stupid fucking questions like that one?

SKI
Well, dMarines are going to help dyou now.

*Lights fade and go out,
one at a time, stage right
to stage left.*

ACT I

SCENE 3

SETTING: *Several weeks later on Ward 2B. A photo of the interior of the ward is projected onto the screen.*

In an arc across the stage from stage right are: BOBBY MAC (now missing the bandage over his eye), JEREMY, and SKI in wheelchairs; DOC MILLER on a stool; a small table holding a rotary dial telephone; MISS BERRY on a stool; a small table; DR. DONNOLLY sitting on a stool; EARL RAY in a wheelchair; an empty wheelchair; and MOOSE in a wheelchair. In front of each seat is a stand for the script.

AT RISE: *As lights come up, one at a time, stage right to stage left, SKI, BOBBY MAC, and JEREMY are laughing.*

SKI
Dyou believe that, Shoff, and I will keese your ass!

BOBBY MAC
Now ain't that some shit! The one thing we all got in common with Shoff is we all have an ass!

EARL RAY
Speak for yourself! I ain't got nothing in common with the noncombat motherfucker. He's just a chicken-shit Navy coward, that's what he is.

JEREMY
We've been over this, Earl. Ain't no way I can change a god-damn thing! You want to hate me for having my arms and legs, go ahead.

EARL RAY
I hate you for a lot of fucking reasons, Shoff. Your girlfriend was right. You ain't got what it takes to be in the Corps. I wouldn't want you near me in a Marine's uniform. I know your kind. You'd probably turn your back and run as soon as it got a little tough. Fuck you, Shoff!

JEREMY
Fuck you, too, Earl! And don't come to me when you need someone to help you stand on your own two feet.

                             EARL RAY
Why, you son-of-a-bitch, I ought to come over there and choke the
living shit out of you!

                             JEREMY
Well come on over if you think you're man enough!

                             EARL RAY
You motherfucker! C'mon, Shoff!
          (*rolls his wheelchair over
           and slams it into Jeremy's*)
Show me what you got!

                             JEREMY
I'm not going to hit you, Earl.

                             EARL RAY
You can't take a man with no legs and only one arm?
          (*shakes his fist*)
What kind of a pussy are you?

                             JEREMY
I'm not going to fight you!

                             EARL RAY
You're a chicken shit! You can't hit a guy with no legs and one
arm? C'mon noncombat motherfucker! Here's your chance!

                             JEREMY (*shouting*)
I ain't going to hit you, Earl!

          *DOC MILLER jumps off his
          stool and jerks EARL RAY's
          wheelchair away from JEREMY,
          pushing it back into its
          place.*

                             DOC MILLER
You stay right there, Earl! Jesus Christ! What's the matter
with you two? Let's see what the hell we've got here. Shit!
          (*stands looking at Jeremy*)
Your leg is going to need stitches, Shoff. How's it feel inside?

                             JEREMY
It's okay, Doc. Sorry. I fell out of bed trying to get the shit
pot off the floor. Earl Ray just came over here to help me.

                             DOC MILLER
What?

                             JEREMY
Well, you know, I dropped it on the floor and I was just trying
to get it when I fell over the edge of the bed. You were really
busy and I --

EARL RAY
Next time, let me get the shit pot off the floor for you.

> *DOC MILLER shakes his head as he walks back and sits on his stool.*

BOBBY MAC
Now ain't that some shit! I thought I left all the bullshit back in Nam.

SKI
Just let eet go, man.

BOBBY MAC
I've let a whole lot worse shit go than this little spat.

EARL RAY
Damn, Shoff, that felt good.

JEREMY
Glad I could help.

EARL RAY
It ain't over, you know.

BOBBY MAC (*laughing*)
Oh, bullshit, Earl, just let it go. Where're you from, Shoff?

JEREMY
Missouri. How 'bout you?

BOBBY MAC
Barlow by-God, North Carolina. My old man's full-blooded Cherokee. Sent me off to the Marines to keep my ass out of trouble. Didn't work. Got into more shit in Nam than anybody. Got to where I didn't even want to go home between tours, but they made me. Wait 'til he sees me now.

JEREMY
You're old man's Cherokee? My great grandmother was Cherokee on my dad's side.

BOBBY MAC
Ain't that some shit! By God, life just got better. I'm lying next to a relative! We'll have us a by-God family reunion right here!

EARL RAY
Yeah. Let's just fucking celebrate.

JEREMY
Your dad coming up anytime soon?

                              BOBBY MAC
Shit. I don't think he even knows I'm in the States. Life ain't
so bad. It's all in how you look at it. Just don't give a shit.

                              JEREMY
I hear you. So you jumped on a live grenade? That takes balls.

                              BOBBY MAC
No balls at all, man. Just did what I was supposed to do.

                              JEREMY
Yeah. Well, not everyone always does what he's supposed to do.

                              BOBBY MAC
It was fucking nothing.

                              JEREMY
Well, I don't think it's nothing.

                              BOBBY MAC
How're you doing down there, Earl Ray?

                              EARL RAY
What's it matter to you?

                              BOBBY MAC
Hey, man. Just trying to check on who I'm sleeping with.

                           EARL RAY (*shouting*)
None of your fucking business, man.

                              MOOSE
Oh, for God's sake. Don't you guys <u>ever</u> shut up down there?

                              EARL RAY
Who the fuck are you? And who made you H-M-F-I-C?

                              MOOSE
I'm Moose Johnson and <u>I</u> made me Head Motherfucker in Charge!

                              EARL RAY
What the fuck kind of name is Moose?

                              MOOSE
A nickname. Got it my first tour in country. We were in thick
brush following an ambush. I heard rustling in the tall grass so
I opened fire with my M60. Shredded a water buffalo into a thousand
pieces. I took shit for a month. Got a tattoo on my left arm
with my new name.

          *BOBBY MAC, JEREMY, SKI,
          and MOOSE all laugh.*

                    EARL RAY
You got a left arm?

                    MOOSE
Not all of it. Lost part of it with the bottom half of my left
leg.

                    EARL RAY
You mobile?

                    MOOSE
Nope. Won't be for a while.

          EARL RAY leans across
          empty wheelchair and
          quietly talks to MOOSE.

                    SKI
               (*to Jeremy*)
Hee'll come around. He's just being a badass. Eet's what he
knows.

                    EARL RAY
Hey, noncombat motherfucker. Moose agreed with me.

                    JEREMY
Yeah? What's that, Earl?

                    EARL RAY
<u>I'm</u> the Head Motherfucker in Charge.

                    JEREMY
I never doubted it, Earl. At least we've got one thing in common.

                    EARL RAY
What's that?

                    JEREMY
We're both motherfuckers.

                    BOBBY MAC
You think?

                    EARL RAY
That new eye of yours is looking good, Bobby Mac. Even I can see
better now that you've got it. In fact, I could even see you had
a catheter bag when they brought you in, this time. Glad to see
that frag didn't get your dick.

                    BOBBY MAC
Yeah, man ain't no way with this club on my hand I could hold
onto that pitcher to piss in, and I couldn't ever find anybody to
hold my dick for me, either! Hey, Shoff. You ever watch that
show, "Laugh-In"?

JEREMY

Yeah, all the time.

BOBBY MAC

Well, you know how those Rowan and Martin guys sign off? Dan Rowan says to Dick Martin, "Say goodnight, Dick," and Dick Martin says, "Goodnight, Dick."

JEREMY

Yeah. They do it every time.

BOBBY MAC
(*looking at his crotch*)

Goodnight, dick.

BOBBY MAC, JEREMY, MOOSE and SKI laugh

Lights begin to fade and go out, one at a time, stage right to stage left...

JEREMY (*sweetly*)

Goodnight, dick!

Halfway across...

SKI (*laughing*)

Gootnight, deek.

As last light goes out...

EARL RAY

Goodnight, assholes.

ACT I

SCENE 4

SETTING: *Sometime later on Ward 2B. A photo of the ward is projected onto the screen behind the actors.*

In an arc across the stage from stage right to stage left are: BOBBY MAC, JEREMY, and SKI in wheelchairs, DOC MILLER on his stool, a small table, a stool where MISS BERRY is sitting, a small table with a certificate and a box with a bow on it, DR. DONNOLLY sitting on a stool, EARL RAY in a wheelchair, an empty chair, and MOOSE in his wheelchair. In front of each seat is a stand for the script.

AT RISE: *The lights come up on each seat in order from stage right to stage left. DOC MILLER is talking to SKI.*

DOC MILLER
Got any special plans for today, Ski?

SKI
I don't, but dwhat do dyou want to know for?

DOC MILLER
Oh, nothing really. Just want to know if you have anything going on.

SKI
Dwhat are you going to do? You can leef my legs alone.

DOC MILLER
I'm not going to do anything with your legs. Well, not right now.

SKI
Thden what do you want weeth me?

EARL RAY
He wants you to sing for him.

JEREMY
Don't look at me, Ski. I don't know what he's talking about.

DOC MILLER
Ski no! Please don't sing.
(MORE)

                              DOC MILLER (CONT'D)
I've heard you and Shoff before, and believe me, I don't need
that. But what I would like is for you to look <u>fine</u>!

                              SKI
Why? Are we going somewhere or do you want to keese me?

                              DOC MILLER
You're not my type, Ski. I prefer American women.

                              SKI
You wouldn't go back to Ameridican women once you had a Roosian
woman.

                              DOC MILLER
Never! Roosian women can't come close to American women.

                              SKI
Just wait. I will set you up with a Roosian woman. A real woman.
She'll take care of your young Ameridican ass.

                              DOC MILLER
She'll have to wait. Right now, I want you to get washed up and
comb your hair.

                              SKI
What the hell eeze going on?

                              JEREMY
I don't know. Better do what Doc says though; he seems pretty
serious about it.

                              EARL RAY
Yeah. Maybe he has an Ameridican woman set up for you.

                              SKI
                         (*grabbing at his crotch*)
Bdring her on, baby! I'll show her really good Roosian time.

                              BOBBY MAC
Maybe he can bring me one, too while he's at it. Ameridican or
Roosian, I don't give a shit!

                    DOC MILLER combs SKI's
                    hair.

                              MISS BARRY
Ski, you look absolutely four-oh.

                              SKI
Thdanks. Meese Berry, what eeze going on?

                              MISS BARRY
I really can't say, Ski. Officer's oath.

I-4-24

> *MISS BARRY quietly exits behind the screen.*

SKI

What the hell eez going on? I don't like theese at all.

DOC MILLER

Nothing at all, Ski.

SKI

Bullsheedt! Dyou had better tell dme dnow.

BOBBY MAC

Better tell him, Doc. He just might make you date that Roosian woman!

DOC MILLER

Okay. Okay. I think we're all ready.

> *MISS BERRY enters the ward with SKI'S POPPA.*

SKI

Poppa!

SKI'S POPPA
(*Embracing Ski*)
Felix, my dboy. Eet has been so dlong. I love dyou my boy! I love dyou! Dyou are home.

SKI

Poppa. Oh, Poppa.

SKI'S POPPA

Look at dyour legs. What eeze all of this? What eeze this thing? They send me letter telling me you weel be fine. You don't look fine to me. Oooh, Felix, this eeze all my fault. If I hadn't let you go. If only I had listened to my heart. I knew some think would be bad. Oh, my boy, I am so sorry. Look what I have done to my only son. Theese doesn't look right to me, my boy. How can dyou come home like this? Eet eez so goot to see you! You must come home now, Momma eez waiting to see you.

SKI

It is so goot to see you, Poppa.
(*the two hug for a moment*)
I must dwait till I can walk again. dThen I can come home.

SKI'S POPPA

I know dyou can't come home right now, my boy, but your Momma can't wait to see you.

SKI

I know Poppa. Soon enough I weel come home.

SKI'S POPPA
I thdink they have a surprise for you, Felix.

SKI
What do you mean? What else could there be?

SKI'S POPPA
I don't know. They just make sure I was here this day.

*MISS BERRY seats SKI'S
POPPA in the empty chair.*

MISS BERRY
You sit over here, Mr. Jamnitzky.

MISS BERRY/DOC MILLER/DR.
DONNOLLY/EARL RAY/BOBBY
MAC/JEREMY/MOOSE,
(*singing*)
From the halls of Montezuuuma to the shores of Tripoli. We will fight our countries baaatles in the air on land and sea.

DR. DONNOLLY
Outstanding! Outstanding!

SKI
What eeze going on here? Dr. Donnolly you don't look right. You being court martialed?

DR. DONNOLLY
Not hardly, Ski. I'm here to let your father know he has a new son.

SKI/SKI'S POPPA (*in unison*)
Dwhat!

DR. DONNOLLY
That's right. Ski, it is with the greatest pride and the deepest honor that I have been selected to present this to you.
   (*taking the certificate
   from the table and reading
   aloud*)
"It is hereby authorized by the President of the United States, Commander in Chief of the Armed Forces, that Felix Dante Jamnitzky, Lance Corporal, United States Marine Corps, from this day and all days forward, is entitled to all inalienable rights guaranteed to every citizen under the Constitution of the United States of America." The President has granted you citizenship. You're a U.S. citizen, Ski!

*A photo of an American
flag replaces the image of
the ward projected on the
screen.*

SKI'S POPPA
(*crying openly and hugging
DR. DONNOLLY*)
My boy is ceetizen? He eez really a ceetizen of America? You are such a great doctor!

SKI
(*holding the certificate
and looking down at his
cast-covered legs*)
Poppa. I am a ceetizen. A U.S. ceetizen. Poppa, eet has all been worth eet.

DOC MILLER
And we're not quite done yet. Got one last surprise for you, Ski, my man!

SKI
Dwhat eeze it now? You going to take me home weeth you?

DOC MILLER
No, it's even better than that.

SKI
Nothing could be better dthan getting out of here.

DOC MILLER
That will come in due time. Right now it's due time for something else.

SKI
Dwhy don't you guys just leef me alone?

EVERYONE ON STAGE
Laughter.

SKI
Am I een some kind of trouble?

DR. DONNOLLY
(*taking the small box from
the table and handing it
to SKI*)
Not at all, young man. We're here to present this to you. The Order of the Purple Heart medal. It's for the sacrifice you made for our nation. Please wear it proudly.

*SKI takes the Purple Heart
medal out of the box. An
image of a Purple Heart
medal replaces the image
of the flag on the screen.*

                        MISS BERRY
It's not every day that I get to be a part of this. Most of the
time it's given before you guys arrive here. Ski, thank you, and
please do wear it with pride. Every one of you, wear yours with
all the pride in the world.

                        SKI'S POPPA
Felix, dmy boy, I must geet home and tell your Momma. She dwill
be so proud. Dwe will come to see you soon. Goot bye, my boy.

                        SKI
Gootbye, Poppa. I can't wait to see you and Momma soon.

            MISS BERRY leads SKI's
            POPPA off the stage as
            EARL RAY pulls his own box
            from his pocket and looks
            at it. He rolls over to
            SKI and shows it to him.

                        EARL RAY
You, me and all the others in here with this, this is who we are.
Take a good look at it, man. Sometimes it feels broken.

                        SKI
Dwhat do dyou mean?

                        EARL RAY
Sometimes it feels like it's broken. You know, like it's all for
nothing.

                        SKI
Dyou are djust feeling Jendeefer, man.

                        EARL RAY
Shit, I've been feeling this way long before that.

                        SKI
Well, I think eet's all about Jendeefer. Dyou should be proud of
dyour Purple Heart.

                        EARL RAY
Yeah, that's what they keep telling me.

                        SKI
Who's dthey?

                        EARL RAY
Those dumb, fucking shrinks they make me go to, who else?

                        SKI
They know what they are talking about. You should leesten to
them.

                    EARL RAY
They don't know a god-damn thing. Trying to tell me my two legs
and arm are worth this little piece of purple and brass. It ain't
why I joined the Corps. I just wanted to be like my old man. Be
a Marine, go to war and come home and just live out my life.
Nobody said I'd come back like this. And they think this Purple
Heart is supposed to make me feel better? They're the ones that
are out of their fucking minds.

                    SKI
Dyou shouldn't feel that way.

                    EARL RAY
Nobody tells me how to feel, Ski. Not even you.

            Lights fade and go out,
            one at a time, stage right
            to stage left.

ACT I

SCENE 5

SETTING: *Another day on Ward 2B. A photo of the ward is projected on the screen.*

In an arc across the stage from stage right are: BOBBY MAC, JEREMY, and SKI in wheelchairs, DOC MILLER on a stool, a small table, an empty stool, a small table, DR. DONNOLLY on a stool, EARL RAY in a wheelchair, an empty space, and MOOSE in his wheelchair. In front of each seat is a stand for the script.

AT RISE: *The lights come on, one at a time, stage right to stage left, as MISS BERRY wheels new patient ROGER to the empty space. ROGER is covered completely in white, including white pajamas and a white balaclava.*

MISS BERRY
(*to ROGER*)
How are you feeling, young man?

ROGER
Not bad, ma'am.

MISS BARRY
I'm Miss Berry. Let me or Doc Miller know if you need anything. Dr. Donnolly will be up later to check on you.

ROGER
Thank you, ma'am.

EARL RAY
Hey Doc. What's the new guy got?

BOBBY MAC
He looks like a giant turtle on its back with his head stuck out.

DOC MILLER
Two broken femurs, two broken arms, cracked skull and busted pelvis, motorcycle. He was home on leave from A-I-T before going to Nam.

SKI
(*laughing at EARL RAY*)
A non-combat moderfucker.

43

                         EARL RAY
                    (*glaring at JEREMY*)
Yeah, but he's a Marine.

                          MOOSE
What difference does it make? Makes no difference, man. We're
all here for the same reason. We got messed up and we gotta get
on with shit, that's all.

                          JEREMY
What's his name?

                        DOC MILLER
Roger George. Just made Lance before he went home.

                          JEREMY
                    (*aside to SKI*)
Well, he may be a Marine, but at least he's noncombat.

                       DR. DONNOLLY
Roger, we need to have a talk about your legs. Your last set of
x-rays shows your two femurs are not healing properly. This body
cast is not working. If we continue as is, your legs will curve
inward. I'm recommending that we put a steel rod in each femur,
just like we did for Jeremy's leg. If you want to walk upright
again, I'm afraid we don't have any other choice.

                          ROGER
I understand sir. When can you do it?

                       DR. DONNOLLY
We'll need to do two separate surgeries at least a week apart.
I'll get them scheduled right away.
                    (*to SKI*))
Good morning, Ski.

                           SKI
Goot morning, sir.

                       DR. DONNOLLY
How do your legs feel inside, Ski?

                           SKI
Not bad, sir. They haven't hurt too badly in a while now.

                       DR. DONNOLLY
That's excellent. You're coming along quite well.

                           SKI
Dthank you. Dr. Donnolly, dyou know those rods you put in Jeremy's
dleg and can put in Roger's, too, to help them heal? Can you put
those things in my dlegs, too?

                              DR. DONNOLLY
I'm sorry, Ski. No one has invented a procedure for shin bones.
You need a hollow bone like the femur for that surgery. But we
do have some really good news. Your legs are doing well enough
we're going to remove the upper half of the casts. We'll remove
them to just below your knees and we'll take the stabilizer bar
out from between your legs, too.

                              SKI
Did dyou guys hear that?

                         EARL RAY/MOOSE/JEREMY/BOBBY
                         MAC cheer.

                              DR. DONNOLLY
And it gets even better. We're going to attach rubber heels to
the bottom of both casts, so we can get you ready to stand up.

                         EARL RAY/MOOSE/JEREMY/BOBBY
                         MAC cheer louder.

                              SKI
dThank you, sir.   dThank you.

                         *DR. DONNOLLY exits behind
                         the screen, with DOC MILLER
                         wheeling SKI after him.
                         When DOC MILLER brings SKI
                         back out, SKI has exchanged
                         his white pants for blue
                         and white striped pajama
                         pants with white coverings
                         below the knees only. He
                         is holding crutches.*

                              DOC MILLER
We're not going to try walking today, Ski. Just get you to stand
up for a few minutes. It's been almost four months since you've
been upright. We'll take it slow. You ready for this?

                              SKI
A dMarine eez aldways ready.

                              DOC MILLER
Alright. Grab these crutches. Here we go.

                         *DOC MILLER tries to help
                         SKI out of his wheelchair
                         with the crutches for
                         support. As SKI tries to
                         stand, he collapses to the
                         ground with his arms over
                         his head.*

                              SKI
Eet got me! Corpsman! My dlegs! My dlegs! Corpsman! Over
here! I've been heet. Corpsman! Corpsman!

                           EARL RAY
It's a flashback, Doc! He's having a flashback!

            DOC Miller cradles SKI in
            his arms.

                           EARL RAY
It's over, Ski. It's over. They can't get you here. It's over,
Ski. The bastards can't get you here.

                          DOC MILLER
                  (*helping SKI back into his*
                       wheelchair)
Oh God, Ski. I'm sorry. I'm so sorry. I should have held on to
you. I'm sorry, Ski. This shot will help. I'm so sorry.

                         DR. DONNOLLY
                   (*rushing onto the ward*)
I got here as fast as I could, Randy. I came as soon as I heard
about Ski. You couldn't have known. You did all you could.

                          DOC MILLER
No, sir. I let him down. I should have known it might happen.
I let him down.

                         DR. DONNOLLY
Don't be so hard on yourself, Randy. No one can predict combat
flashbacks. They just happen. We all do the best we can.

                     DOC MILLER (*weeping*)
Yeah, I guess so.

                         DR. DONNOLLY
How are feeling, Ski?

                              SKI
Nawt too bad.

                         DR. DONNOLLY
Ski, we need to take some X-rays right away. I have to see if
anything serious is going on in there. That means we need to
lift your legs up a bit. You ready to let us take a look?

                           EARL RAY
A Marine is always ready.

            DOC MILLER pushes SKI
            behind the screen, with
            DR. DONNOLLY following
            them.

SKI (*groggily*)
Damn dright. A dMarine eez always ready.

> *After a pause, DR. DONNOLLY slowly returns.*

DR. DONNOLLY
It's SKI's right leg, men. It was damaged pretty badly from his fall. He was bleeding internally and it couldn't wait. We had to amputate. I wanted to tell you myself so you'd be ready when he gets here.

> *DOC MILLER slowly pushes SKI back into his place on the ward. The white "cast" on SKI's right leg is now covered by black from the knee down.*

DOC MILLER
I'm so sorry, Ski. I'll make it up to you. I will. Somehow. I will.

> *EARL RAY rolls over to SKI's wheelchair and takes his hand.*

EARL RAY (*sadly*)
Welcome to the club, my friend. Welcome to the club.

> *The lights fade and go out, one at a time, stage right to stage left.*

ACT I

SCENE 6

SETTING: *Several days later on Ward 2B. A photo of the interior of the ward is projected onto the screen.*

In an arc across the stage from stage right are: BOBBY MAC, JEREMY, and SKI in wheelchairs; DOC MILLER on a stool; a small table holding a rotary dial telephone; MISS BERRY on a stool; a small table; an empty stool; EARL RAY in a wheelchair; an empty wheelchair and MOOSE in his wheelchair. In front of each seat is a stand for the script.

AT RISE: *As lights come up, one at a time, stage right to stage left, SKI, BOBBY MAC, and JEREMY are laughing.*

DOC MILLER
(*into phone*)
Hello. Doc Miller, Ward 2B. Yes, just a sec. Hey, Earl! It's for you.

EARL RAY
Who's calling me?

DOC MILLER
Don't know. She wouldn't say.

BOBBY MAC
Hot damn! I'll bet it's that Roosian woman.

SKI
Give him the phone, Doc!

DOC MILLER carries the phone down to EARL RAY.

EARL RAY
No need to leave it, Doc. This won't take long.
(*into phone*)
Hello?
(*pause*)
Oh, hi, Jen, I thought it might be you.
(*pause*)
No need to be sorry. You didn't do anything anyone else wouldn't have done.

(MORE)

I-6-35

                    EARL RAY (CONT'D)
          (*pause*)
I didn't mean that.
          (*pause*)
Yeah, I've been doin' a lot of thinking, too. I'm not sure trying again just now is a good idea.
          (*dropping the phone*)
Son of a bitch!

          DOC MILLER picks up the
          phone and hands it back
          to EARL RAY.

                    EARL RAY
          (*into phone*)
Sorry, Babe.
          (*pause*)
Yes, I guess I did call you, Babe.
          (*pause*)
I don't think coming to see me again is a good idea, Jen.
          (*pause*)
You know why, Jen. I need a lot of time. A lot more time.
          (*pause*)
Yeah, I'm getting your letters, Jen. I just don't feel like writing.
          (*pause*)
I can't call you, not for a while.
          (*pause*)
Okay, Jen. Okay. Bye.

                    SKI
Dyou are a dlucky guy, Earl. She eez a special woman, dyou know. Dyou should call her back.

                    EARL RAY
Yeah, some day. Some day when I'm feeling lucky. Not today.

                    MISS BERRY
You really should call her back someday, Earl.

                    EARL RAY
Yeah. Maybe, someday.

                    MISS BERRY
Okay then, everyone, let's get this inspection over with. It's too bad Roger's down in Post-Op and has to miss the excitement, because in that full-body cast, at least I'd be able to count on <u>one</u> of you to behave himself. The rest of you, I'm not so sure about. I know it's asking a lot, but <u>please</u> be on your best behavior today. This shouldn't take long and everything will be back to normal. Wish me luck. I'll be back up here with the brass in a few minutes.

> *MISS BERRY exits behind the screen.*

EARL RAY

Hey, Doc.

DOC MILLER

Yeah, what is it, Earl?

EARL RAY

We know the brass is coming up, but who is it?

DOC MILLER

This is the <u>big</u> guy. The admiral from Norfolk headquarters.

SKI

I've never seen an admeeral. I don't think they are allowed in Nam!

EARL RAY

Non-combat motherfuckers, all of 'em.

JEREMY

Just like me.

EARL RAY

No, not quite like you. At least you went through boot camp. These guys wouldn't know a boot if it kicked 'em in the ass.

BOBBY MAC

Ain't that some shit. We must be real important if an admiral is coming.

EARL RAY

Yeah. We're supposed to think they give a shit.

> *The ADMIRAL and MISS BERRY come in and walk down the line of wheelchairs. The ADMIRAL stops when he gets to EARL RAY, who is staring down at his left half-leg. None of the patients are saluting. Only EARL RAY is singled out.*

ADMIRAL

Where's your salute, young man?

> *EARL RAY doesn't move.*

ADMIRAL

I said, where's your salute, young man?

EARL RAY straightens up as much as he can, and salutes with his right hand. He never looks at the ADMIRAL.

                    JEREMY
     (*to the ADMIRAL*)
Are you shittin' me?

                SKI/EARL RAY/BOBBY MAC
Holy shit!

                    ADMIRAL
     (*to JEREMY*)
What is it that you have to say to me, young man?

                    JEREMY
With all due respect sir, I think <u>you're</u> the one who should be saluting <u>him</u>.

                    ADMIRAL
What's your name, sailor?

                    JEREMY
Shoff, sir. Jeremy Shoff.

                ADMIRAL (*furiously*)
You're up for Captain's Mast, Shoff, as soon you're able.

The ADMIRAL storms off the ward with MISS BERRY following him. When the doors close behind them, Ward 2B erupts in cheers.

                    SKI
Holy shdit! What deed you do, man?

                  EARL RAY
That was fucking unbelievable, Shoff!

                    JEREMY
I can't believe he would come in here and expect you guys to salute him. Who the hell does he think he is?

                  BOBBY MAC
Shoff, you are beaucoup dinky dow! You're a crazy motherfucker! You got balls as big as that brass's ribbon rack!

                    JEREMY
I wouldn't know, man. Right now, I can't find 'em.

MOOSE

You are in deep shit, my friend.

EARL RAY

Shoff, you're all right by me. Non-combat motherfucker or not, I can't believe you did that.

SKI
(giving JEREMY a salute)
I dsalute d<u>you</u>, Shoff!

JEREMY

Thanks, Ski, but I've got my ass in big trouble and it's Miss Berry I'm worried about. I don't know what she's going to say to me.

BOBBY MAC

Ain't that some shit! Beaucoup dinky Dow, Shoff! You're a crazy mother fucker!
(farting loudly.)
Keep talking admiral, we'll find you.

Everyone laughs.

MOOSE

Shoff is right, you know. We don't have to salute those bastards! What are they going to do? Send us to Nam?

EARL RAY/SKI/BOBBY MAC

Damn right! Hell yes!

MISS BERRY returns to the ward and stage whispers in JEREMY's ear.

MISS BERRY

I will deny that I ever said this, but, thank you, Jeremy.
(to everyone)
Well! Now that <u>that's</u> over with, anyone going to P-T, make sure you wrap those <u>limbs</u> tight. We don't want any swollen limbs in the morning.

DOC MILLER

Yeah, the guys down in physical therapy won't be too happy if you're a mess when you come back tomorrow.

EARL RAY

What do they care? Those guys are like gorillas, anyway. Swollen stumps don't slow them down.

MOOSE
(flexing the muscle in his
 left arm)
It takes gorillas to make gorillas.

                                    SKI
They push hard, but they can't push us hard enough. Eet feels
goot to be lifting weights again.

                                MISS BERRY
That's the attitude, you guys. The faster you get stronger, the
quicker you can transfer to the rehab wards and then on your way
home. Out there, you'll be on your own. All you will have is
each other.

                                DOC MILLER
If I ever get into a fight, I want you guys on my side.
                          (*everyone chuckles*)
We'll see you in the morning.

                     MISS BARRY and DOC MILLER
                      exit behind the screen.

                                 EARL RAY
C'mon Shoff. Get that rickshaw of yours and let's go have a smoke.

                                  JEREMY
It's raining out, man. Haven't you noticed?

                                 EARL RAY
We ain't going out. We're going to the room.

                       JEREMY begins to fidget
                         and wring his hands.

                                BOBBY MAC
Relax, Shoff. We ain't taking you to the fucking gallows.

                                  JEREMY
Don't be so sure. I've heard you and the others share stories
about the solarium. It's sacred ground for you guys. I don't
belong in there. Dr. Donnolly made it off limits to anyone not a
patient on 2B. And you guys made it off limits to noncombat
motherfuckers like me.

                                 EARL RAY
If we invite you, you're going in.

                                  JEREMY
                            (*wiping his brow*)
I don't know, Earl. It's not right for me to join you guys in
there. I don't deserve to be in that room with you guys. Shit, I
don't deserve to be on the same ward with you.

                                BOBBY MAC
Bullshit, Shoff. Don't you dare fucking say no to us. Hey, Ski,
Shoff's coming. You want to join us?

SKI
I dwouldn't meesse eet for nothing. Somebody go call down to the rehabs and get Big Al to come up. He dwon't want to meese this.

> *Stage lights fade and go out, one at a time, stage right to stage left.*

ACT I

SCENE 7

SETTING: *The Solarium, late evening. A photo of a wall of glass windows is projected on the screen.*

In an arc across the stage from stage right are: BOBBY MAC, JEREMY, SKI, and EARL RAY in their wheelchairs, an empty space, and MOOSE in his wheelchair. In front of each seat is a stand for the script.

AT RISE: *As the lights come up, one at a time, from stage right to stage left, they are all talking.*

MOOSE
Did you guys call down to Q ward for Big Al?

BIG AL
Did I hear my name?

BIG AL rolls in and takes his place in the half circle.

MOOSE
Man, that didn't take long. Glad you could join us.

BIG AL
I wouldn't miss this for the world.

EARL RAY
How's everything out on the rehabs, Big Al?

BIG AL
Same old shit, Earl. Be glad when you get out there. I need somebody to beat at Spades.

EARL RAY
You couldn't beat me in a chair race. I haven't heard when they're moving me back out, but when they do, I'll race you down the ramps.

BIG AL
You got a deal.

EARL RAY
(flexing his right arm)
And I don't need a head start either.

                          BIG AL
I wouldn't have it any other way.

                          BIG AL
                       (to Jeremy)
Hey, Shoff. Earl Ray says you don't like being called a non-combat
motherfucker. Don't blame you. Earl Ray should worry more about
himself instead of looking around at what everybody else has or
doesn't have. Ain't that right, Earl Ray?

                         EARL RAY
I'm the one that said we ought to bring him in here, ain't I?
Don't mean shit to me anymore what anybody's done. Nothing means
shit to me anymore.

                           SKI
Dwhat about Jendeefer?

                         EARL RAY
What about <u>Jendeefer</u>? Jennifer ain't shit either. I'm just
going to get me a whore to live with when I get out of here.
Somebody that doesn't know shit about me and doesn't want to know.

                          MOOSE
Okay. Okay. Let's save it for later. Big Al, did you bring
that care package from your buddies in Nam?

                          BIG AL
Absolutely! And a surprise! I brought a bottle of Jack!

           *BIG AL pulls a bottle of
           Jack Daniels from under
           his pajama top and a small
           bundle from behind his
           back and opens it. From
           the bundle, he pulls out a
           couple of Thai sticks, a
           short letter, and a couple
           of Polaroid pictures. As
           the guys pass the pictures
           and joints around, EARL
           RAY opens the Jack Daniels,
           takes a swig and hands two
           of the photos to JEREMY.*

                         EARL RAY
Ain't that a pretty sight? Take it in Shoff. Take as much time
as you need, man. You look at it long enough you may not give a
shit either?

           *JEREMY looks, hands the
           pictures to SKI, then takes
           a swig of the Jack and
           hangs his head.*

EARL RAY

You wanted to be here, Shoff. If you don't like it, now's your chance to leave.

JEREMY

I ain't leaving, Earl. A couple of pictures with dead people ain't going to make me go. I just don't want you to hate my guts. I can't change who I am and what's happened.

EARL RAY

I don't hate your guts, Shoff. I just hate who you are. I hate every motherfucker out there. So don't think you're so special. If I didn't want you in here, believe me, you wouldn't be in here.

JEREMY

You guys don't know what it means for me to be in this room.

SKI

Yes, dwe do. We just weesh you dwere a dMarine.

MOOSE

So. We've talked it over Shoff. We think you're all right for a non-combat motherfucker. We all agree. You're in here because we want you in here. Shoff, we're making you an honorary Marine!

JEREMY sits up straight and smiles.

EARL RAY

Just because you stood up to that admiral doesn't mean you're one of us, Shoff. It just means we don't mind having you around.

JEREMY

I gave up my chance to be one of you a long time ago. But if it's all right with you guys, when I get out to the rehabs, I'll get me a tattoo-Honorary U.-S.-M.-C.

EARL RAY

I'll go with you and make sure it ain't too big. And it can't be where anyone can see it.

JEREMY

I wouldn't care if it was on the top of my head.

SKI

Dyou see. dThat is why we like you.

BOBBY MAC

Now, ain't that some shit! We got us a genuine honorary by-God fuckin' Marine! And a relative to boot! Don't get no better than this man!

> JEREMY passes BOBBY MAC
> the bottle of Jack and
> BOBBY MAC takes a big swig.

EARL RAY

Don't get too cocky, Shoff. You'll always be a noncombat motherfucker. So don't forget it. Bobby Mac, hand me that Jack.

> The guys pass around the
> Jack Daniels and there is
> a quiet pause. EARL RAY
> takes a big drink from the
> bottle.

EARL RAY

It's happening you know.

MOOSE

What's that?

EARL RAY

People are beginning to hate us.

MOOSE

Ain't a damn thing we can do about it.

EARL RAY

Yeah, but how can they hate a guy with no legs? What the fuck do they know?

MOOSE

Fuck 'em. We don't owe them shit anyway.

BOBBY MAC

Ain't that some shit. Their day will come.

EARL RAY

You think they ever think they might owe us something? Fuck no they don't. They're spitting on our guys coming home for Christ's sake!

MOOSE

Take it easy, Earl. You don't want to get worked up over those assholes.

BOBBY MAC

Moose is right, Earl. They ain't shit and won't ever be shit to us.

EARL RAY

If I had my legs, I'd track every one of them down and kill those fucking long hairs with my bare hand.

MOOSE
If I had my leg and my arm, I'd just go home and start all over.

EARL RAY
You mean you'd join the Corps and go back to Nam? That's bullshit.

MOOSE
No. I didn't say that. I said I'd start all over again. Just like I'm going to when I get my arm and leg and get out of here.

EARL RAY
It ain't the same.

MOOSE
I know it ain't the same. But it's what we got and we got to get used to it.

EARL RAY
(*points at his left stump*)
This is what we got, huh? I'm supposed to feel lucky because I've got my cock and that cheap fucking Purple Heart? Bull shit.

MOOSE
It's what we got, Earl. That and each other. You think I can do this alone? We all need someone's help, someone we can count on.

EARL RAY
I don't need anybody's help.

MOOSE
That ain't that what the Corps drilled into our thick heads.

EARL RAY
That's different.

MOOSE
No difference at all, Earl. Remember your first real combat? Man, I do. All the rah-rah in the world and I was still scared shitless. Well, I'm scared shitless now, my friend.

BOBBY MAC
Got to look at what you have, Earl. Not at what you used to have.

EARL RAY
You're right, Moose. Ain't nothing different about any of it. But I did the right thing, you know.

MOOSE
You know you did, Earl. All of us did.

EARL RAY
Yeah, but Jesus, look at me. You know, I still can't believe it. If I could only go back, get another chance, like it never happened.

MOOSE

It's okay, Earl. We all feel that way sometimes.

EARL RAY

What the fuck am I going to do? A man with no legs? One arm? You call this a man?

MOOSE

You're a whole lot more of a man than anybody, Earl. You're more of a man than any fucking long hair out there. You got to be proud of what you did in Nam.

EARL RAY

Yeah, well, fuck the war. And fuck the medals. Big fucking deal. Pieces of cloth and cheap tin that don't mean shit. They can't give me back my arm, my legs god dammit.

SKI

Dyou should be proud of dyour medals. Dyou deed --

EARL RAY

I know what I did. I killed enough of those fuckers to protect this country for a century. And what do I get? Salute the brass. Sit tall in your wheelchair. Be proud of what you did for your country. The Marine Corps builds men. Semper Fi. Bullshit. Simple fucking bullshit.

SKI

No matter dwhat, Earl, you got us.

EARL RAY

It was the right thing to do, right? What else could I have done? It's what I wanted, to be a Marine. Now, I just count my blessings. At least I have my cock. Both eyes are perfect, right? No shrapnel to the head or face. Man, how fuckin' lucky can I be? I'm still alive, right? So what's my bitch? Fuck the legs. Fuck the arm. Semper Fi, my ass. The Marine Corps builds stumps.

MOOSE

It's okay, Earl. This is life now. Anything you want, you know we're here.

EARL RAY

You think it's that easy, huh?

MOOSE

No. It ain't easy, Earl. Not for any of us.

EARL RAY

It's real easy for the non-combat motherfucker. Ain't that right, Shoff?

MOOSE

We all got shit to deal with.

                              JEREMY
It's okay, Moose. There's nothing I can say. Not to Earl, not
to you, or Ski, not to anybody. But if I had it to do over again,
I probably wouldn't be here right now. Who knows what would have
happened? What's done is done, Earl. For what it's worth, backing
out of the Marines was the most chicken-shit thing I've ever done.
And I'll regret it for the rest of my life. But no matter what
you think about me, you can count on me anytime.

                             EARL RAY
Count on you? For what? To piss me off? To remind me of all
the noncombat motherfuckers out there? To remind me how lucky I
am? Ski keeps telling me how lucky I am. You're the lucky one,
Shoff. Lucky I didn't kill you. Lucky you got both arms. And
lucky you've got your legs. On the day you <u>walk</u> out of here,
Shoff, stop and think how lucky you are.

                              JEREMY
I wouldn't call it luck, Earl.

                             EARL RAY
Then what do you call it?   Fate?

                              JEREMY
No, I call it shame.

          *Lights fade and go out,
          one a time, stage right to
          stage left.*

ACT I

SCENE 8

SETTING: *The patients' last day on Ward 2B. A photo of the ward is projected on the screen.*

In an arc across the stage from stage right are: BOBBY MAC, an empty wheelchair, and SKI in his wheelchair, DOC MILLER on a stool, a small table, MISS BERRY on a stool, a small table, DR. DONNOLLY on a stool, EARL RAY, ROGER, and MOOSE in their wheelchairs. In front of each seat is a stand for the script.

AT RISE: *As the lights come up, one at a time, stage right to stage left, DOC MILLER walks over to SKI.*

MOOSE
Hey, Doc. You're sure looking damn sharp. You getting ready for a big night out?

DOC MILLER
Nope. It's just another Friday night for me. Besides, with you guys graduating to the rehab ward, I'm taking two weeks' leave starting tomorrow. Remember? Got an early flight.

SKI
No one deserves eet more than you.

DOC MILLER
Well, I don't know about that, but I understand they're sending you guys all out to the rehabs before I get back. You've done great. And remember. Once you're out there, you have to take care of each other.

ROGER
Ain't none of us could have made it without you.

DOC MILLER
Thanks. I know I couldn't have made it through some of the days if it hadn't been for you guys, too. If I'm lucky, maybe I can look you guys up when I get back.

EARL RAY
What do you mean when you get back? How much time off did they give you?

DOC MILLER
You know, the usual two weeks.

BOBBY MAC
Give <u>me</u> two weeks leave and you'll never see my ass in here again.

Everyone laughs.

EARL RAY
Make sure you come out to the rehabs and find us when you get back.

DOC MILLER
Oh, I think you will all be long gone and home by then, my friends.

SKI
Dwhat do you mean, Doc?

DOC MILLER
I got my orders. I volunteered and I'm going to Vietnam. I owe it to you, Ski. I'm going to Nam.

SKI
Sawnoffabeetch.

Everyone sits quiet. EARL RAY looks around the ward. DOC MILLER shakes everyone's hand, says goodbye and exits.

DR. DONNOLLY
Your being here has been a special time for all of us, not just for Randy. It takes a special person to do what you guys have done, and it has been my honor to be your doctor and surgeon. As I told each one of you, you're healing has only begun. Don't miss a day of physical therapy and if you do nothing else, keep every single appointment with your psychiatrists. They're going to help you get through the next few months and ready to go home.

SKI
Thdank you, Dr. Donnolly. Dyou are the best.

DR. DONNOLLY
(*shaking SKI's hand*)
Thank you, Ski. And let me say again, welcome to America.

SKI
(*sitting up tall in his wheelchair*)
My Poppa is so proud of dyou. He still thinks dyou did it.

DR. DONNOLLY
It was one of my most treasured moments with you guys. I'll never forget it.

MOOSE
We'll give Ski another celebration once we're all out on the rehabs. Big Al and Jeremy are already out there making plans.

BOBBY MAC
Great! We'll have that by-God family reunion, too!

EARL RAY
You won't think it's so great once we get out there.

BOBBY MAC
We'll just have to make it great then. C'mon, guys. Let's get out of here and make room for the incoming.

DR. DONNOLLY
You men can come back up here anytime. We would be honored to see you.

BOBBY MAC
(*spreading his eyelids,
displaying his glass eye*)
I'll keep an eye out on these guys for you.
(*laughter*)

MISS BERRY
(*putting her hand on EARL
RAY's shoulder*)
It's been a long journey to this point. You're going to need each other on the rehab ward. Take care of each other.
(*choking up*)
I'm going to miss all of you.

ROGER
Even me, Miss Berry?

MISS BERRY (*laughing*)
No, Roger. Not you. You're not going anywhere just yet. That's just wishful thinking on your part.

ROGER (*laughing*)
Just thought I'd ask. You never know what the gorillas might be able to do to rehab a man in a full-body cast. And you know more bodies will be coming in soon, to fill all the rest of these beds.

*The lights fade and go
out, one at a time, stage
right to stage left. As
last light goes out...*

EARL RAY
When is this shit ever going to stop?

END OF ACT I

ACT II

SCENE 1

SETTING: *Q Ward. A photo of the hospital is projected onto a screen behind the actors. A full-length mirror stands beside the screen.*

In an arc across the stage from stage right to stage left are: BOBBY MAC in his wheelchair, a wheelchair for JEREMY, SKI in his wheelchair, a stool, a footlocker, and EARL RAY, BIG AL and MOOSE in their wheelchairs. All the Marines are wearing their non-dress, USMC khaki uniforms. Assorted mechanical arms and legs hang on the sides of the wheelchairs. In front of each seat is a stand for the script.

AT RISE: *As the lights come up on each seat in order from stage right to stage left, JEREMY comes in wearing his white Navy uniform, limping and carrying a half-full sea bag.*

BOBBY MAC
Well, looky here! My blood relative all dressed up and playing Navy! I didn't recognize you Shoff. You getting ready for that by-God family reunion? Or is that admiral after your ass?

JEREMY
I only wear it when I have to, Bobby. And the admiral probably is after my ass.

SKI
dWhat do you mean, you wear it only when you have to?

JEREMY
They gave me a temporary light-duty assignment in Special Services. An unbelievable desk job.

MOOSE
They may as well make it permanent. You still got a lot of P.-T. left.

JEREMY
Yeah. I'm going to stay here with you guys for as long as I can. My first medical review board gave me three more months here.

SKI
dWhat do you do in Special Services?

JEREMY
You won't believe it. I'm in charge of the party desk! Well, that's what I call it. This is the biggest personnel mistake the Navy ever made. But for you guys, it's a miracle.

BIG AL
You're in charge of a party desk? We've hit the jackpot!

JEREMY
You got that right. It's clam bakes, picnics, and Welcome Home parties sponsored by local V.-F.-Ws, American Legion posts, and even a brewery.

BOBBY MAC
Well, when do we start?

JEREMY
Not for a couple of weeks. We're just now getting things lined up. Man is it good to see you guys. They sent me to M Ward while I've been waiting for you to get out here to the rehabs. Mind if I bunk here?

EARL RAY
You got two good arms and two good legs, Shoff, so get your ass on the top bunk next to the shithouse. I got the bottom bunk next to yours and Big Al has the bottom bunk next to me. If you don't like where we put you, then move back to the other ward.

JEREMY
This is fine with me, Earl. And the shithouse doesn't bother me either.

EARL RAY
We didn't put you there to piss you off. We want you close to the shithouse in case one of us needs you to wipe his ass.

JEREMY
Don't count on it.

EARL RAY
I knew I couldn't count on you, Shoff. Not even to wipe my ass.

JEREMY
Okay, Earl. I'll wipe your ass if you need me to. But don't expect me to pull you out of the shitter if you fall in.

EARL RAY
Fuck you, Shoff. Look around you, man. We're all in the shithouse already.

                    JEREMY
This ain't so bad. It's better than 2B.

                    EARL RAY
Says you. We've got no morphine out here.

                    JEREMY
Is the pain that bad, Earl?

                    EARL RAY
It's always that bad. Welcome to Q.

                    MOOSE
Welcome to Q, Shoff! You got that bunk because we don't want someone we don't know sleeping too close to us. Besides, you can stand watch over this end of the ward from up there.

                    JEREMY
No one gets past that you don't want to get past.

                    MOOSE
Ski has the bunk over there and Big Al and Bobby Mac have those two bunks. Glad to have you here, Shoff.

                    BOBBY MAC
Just one big happy family! Maybe we can finally have that by-God family reunion!

                    EARL RAY
May as well make yourself at home, Shoff. We're going to be in this shit hole for a while.
                        (*grabbing his three
                        prosthetic limbs*)
I'm taking a piss today.

                    BIG AL
You take a piss every day.

                    EARL RAY
This time I'm standing up. I'm tired of sitting down to piss like a girl. I think I'm ready.

                    BOBBY MAC
Go for it man.

                    EARL RAY
                        (*wheeling himself behind
                        the screen*)
I need you guys nearby. Just in case.

                    BIG AL
We're right here, Earl, if you need us.

> *On the way behind the screen, EARL RAY looks in the mirror next to it. After a moment, he comes back out and looks at the mirror again.*

EARL RAY

Told you, Shoff.

JEREMY

I never doubted it, Earl.

EARL RAY

Dumb, fucking shrinks. I'd like to smash that damn thing. I know it was their idea to put a mirror where you have to pass by it to get to the head. No one else would'a done it.

> *PAPPY, in a Coast Guard uniform, enters Q ward from stage right. He is carrying a duffle bag in his right hand; his left hand and forearm are covered in white. He looks bewildered and confused.*

JEREMY

How's it going?

PAPPY

Doing okay. I'm supposed to bunk here for a couple of weeks. They sent me out here and told me to find an empty bunk. Is this the right place?

BOBBY MAC

Well, hell yeah! Anybody that's got a four-year stripe on his sleeve is welcome on Q! You look like you just seen a fucking ghost! C'mon on in. Grab any bunk as long as it ain't mine.

PAPPY

Thanks. Is anywhere okay?

MOOSE

You got two full legs and both arms, you take a top bunk.

PAPPY

That's not a problem.
> (*putting down his bag, PAPPY sits on the stool*)

MOOSE (*pointing*)

Your name tag says Richards. What's your first name?

                              PAPPY
Sonny.

                              MOOSE
Well, Sonny Richards, what kind of uniform is that you're wearing,
and what are you doing here?

                              PAPPY
                        (*looking down at the floor*)
It's Coast Guard. I busted my hand in a training exercise so
they sent me here for a couple of weeks of P.-T.

                              EARL RAY
You're fucking Coast Guard? Jesus Christ, we got us one more noncombat motherfucker. You're in a world of shit. Just ask Shoff.
And if they said you'll be here two weeks, you'll probably be
here a couple of months.

                              PAPPY
Uh, I don't have to bunk here, guys, if it's going to be a problem.

                              BOBBY MAC
Bullshit! We don't really give a shit what you do. You're in
here now and that's that.

                              SKI
Don't dmind Earl. He'll be okay weeth it.

                              PAPPY
You sure it's okay? I can bunk somewhere else.

                              BOBBY MAC
You've come to the right place, my friend. Let me give you a
hand with that duffel bag.

                              PAPPY
Sure, uh, thanks.

                        *BOBBY MAC takes off his
                        rubber hand and tosses it
                        to PAPPY. PAPPY grabs the
                        hand and stares at it.*

                              MOOSE
Give me that damn thing.
                        (*MOOSE grabs the hand and
                        the Marines start tossing
                        it back and forth.*)

                              EARL RAY
Why the hell did you come through the side doors? You think you
could sneak in here? Maybe steal something?

PAPPY
No, not at all. I drove out here from the front gate. They said go to Q, so I found Q Ward marked on the side of the building and well, that's where I parked my car.

SKI/JEREMY/BIG AL/MOOSE/ROGER
You what!

PAPPY
Yeah, I drove. My car's sitting right outside.

BOBBY MAC, JEREMY, SKI, and MOOSE make their ways to stage right and look out, then return to their wheelchairs.

MOOSE
Son of a bitch! Our prayers have been answered.

BOBBY MAC
A genuine by-God limousine if I ever saw one!

BIG AL
Come on in. We've got just the bunk for you!

EARL RAY
A car? So what. Doesn't mean shit. You're letting him in here because he has a car? Another noncombat motherfucker.

PAPPY
Really guys. I can bunk somewhere else.

BOBBY MAC
Not unless you leave us that car, you ain't. Do you know how far it is to the front gate? It takes a guy with both legs twenty minutes.

EARL RAY
(*pointing to JEREMY*)
Yeah, just ask Shoff. Ain't that right noncombat motherfucker.

JEREMY
(*looking straight at EARL RAY*)
Yeah, that's right, Earl. If it makes you feel any better, I'll take a wheelchair the next time and race you to the front.

EARL RAY
(*flexing his right arm muscle*)
Shit, you couldn't beat me with both arms. Remember this?

II-1-57

JEREMY
(*swallowing hard*)
Yeah. I remember it. Don't' get any ideas. I'm never going to hit you, Earl.

EARL RAY
You're still a chicken shit Navy coward.

MOOSE
Okay, okay. I thought we left that shit back on 2B. You two settle this some other time, huh? We'll take a vote. All in favor of a Coasty staying on Q, raise your hand if you got one. Otherwise, raise a stump.

Everyone but EARL RAY votes to keep PAPPY on the ward.

MOOSE
It's settled. Welcome to Q, Sonny.

PAPPY
Thanks guys. I'll try to stay out of the way.

EARL RAY
Yeah. Welcome to Q. Just keep your noncombat ass away from me.

MOOSE
He'll come around, Sonny. How long have you been in the Coast Guard?

PAPPY
Just over seven years.

BOBBY MAC
Shit man, you don't look old enough to be out of high school.

PAPPY
Yeah, I'll be twenty-eight my next birthday.

BOBBY MAC
No shit! You're an old bastard! By God, we'll just call you Pappy! Pappy the sailor man.

BIG AL
Well, Pappy, you won't mind being our taxi once in a while, will you?

PAPPY
Well, sure. As long as I'm around, I'll take you guys anywhere.

MOOSE
Perfect, Pappy, this bunk right over here is yours. Welcome to Q.

                    SKI
dJust another beautiful day in paradise!

                    BOBBY MAC
Sure as hell beats Nam.

                    EARL RAY
Yeah, well, it was Nam that put us in this shithole.

                    MOOSE
This ain't so bad, Earl. It won't be long before we all get out
of here and head home.

                    EARL RAY
What the fuck is home? I'm never going home. Ain't shit in
Florida anymore.

                    SKI
Are you steel getting letters from Jendeefer?

                    EARL RAY
Yeah, I'm still getting letters from <u>Jendeefer</u>.

                    SKI
dWhat does she have to say?

                    EARL RAY
How the hell would I know? I haven't read any of them.

                    SKI
dWhat the hell do dyou do weeth them, Earl?

                    EARL RAY
I just toss 'em in my locker.

                    MOOSE
They're in your locker? Unopened?

                    EARL RAY
That's what I said, didn't I?

                    SKI
dYou are a lucky guy, Earl. dYou should read them. dYou should
call her someday.

                    EARL RAY
Yeah, like I said before. Maybe someday when I'm feeling lucky.

                    MOOSE
That day will come, Earl. The day you get out of here will be
your lucky day. None of us can stay in here forever.

                    EARL RAY
Maybe I won't make it out of here. Maybe I don't want to.

MOOSE
C'mon, Earl, that's no way to talk.

EARL RAY
The way I see it, I've got two choices. Live the rest of my life stuck in this fucking chair, or finish what the land mine didn't do.

MOOSE
Shit, Earl, you can come live with me.

EARL RAY
You're really funny, Moose.

MOOSE
I'm not being funny, my friend. Think about it, will you?

EARL RAY
Yeah. I'll think about it. Got nowhere else to go.

MOOSE
(*looking at SKI*)
Hey, Ski, how's that new plastic leg fitting you?

SKI (*grinning*)
Like a glove.

BOBBY MAC
Shit. If your leg fits like a glove, then my hand fits like a shoe!

Everyone laughs.

MOOSE
How about you, Big Al? You're standing tall in that rocking horse you use sometimes, my friend.

BIG AL
Giddy up! I'm ready to ride.

JEREMY
That sounds like a plan. Tell you what, Big Al, how about you and me go out and find a place to have a few beers?

BIG AL
Yeah, you and me, and this anchor on my ass.

JEREMY
You don't need that rocking horse, you got me.

BIG AL
What do you mean?

JEREMY
Just what I said. Get off that high horse of yours and let's go.

> *JEREMY bends down. BIG AL grabs JEREMY around the neck. JEREMY stands up, lifting BIG AL onto his back. BIG AL is smiling from ear to ear.*

JEREMY
Climb on, Big Al. We're going places!

> *JEREMY and BIG AL head toward the side door.*

JEREMY
We'll head north to the first street and take a look around. This is a Navy base. There has to be a bar nearby.

BIG AL
I go where you go.

> *JEREMY and BIG AL exit stage right.*

BIG AL (O.S.)
Oh, look! There one is, Shoff! The Rainbow Bar and Grille.

JEREMY (O.S.)
Hell of a name for a bar, ain't it?

BIG AL (O.S.)
Doesn't matter to me if they <u>name</u> it Hell. Just get me inside!

> *JEREMY and BIG AL laugh.*

> *Lights fade and go out, one at a time, stage right to stage left.*

ACT II

SCENE 2

SETTING: *The Rainbow Bar and Grille. A photo of the interior of a neighborhood bar is projected onto a screen behind the actors.*

The wheelchairs have been removed. Three bar-height round tables, each with three stools facing the front, are spaced across the stage. JEREMY in his Navy white uniform and BIG AL in his USMC non-dress khaki uniform sit at the table stage right. EVA, wearing a robe over hotpants and a tube top, is sitting at the table on stage left. On each table is a stand for the script.

AT RISE: *As the lights come up on each seat in order from stage right to stage left, BAR PATRON is carrying JEREMY and BIG AL a pitcher of beer and two glasses on a tray.*

BAR PATRON
Let me get these for you.

JEREMY/BIG AL
Thanks, man! We sure appreciate it.

BAR PATRON sits with EVA at the table stage left. They talk quietly for a moment as JEREMY and BIG AL drink and BAR PATRON nods his head towards JEREMY and BIG AL.

EVA gets up and dances her way over to sit down next to BIG AL. She flicks a finger nail at the hospital band on BIG AL's left wrist and holds BIG AL by the hand.

EVA
Nice to have you guys here. What're your names?

                           BIG AL
                    (*a little nervous*)
I'm Al. Big Al. Everyone calls me Big Al. This is Shoff.

                            EVA
                    (*glancing at where BIG AL's
                     legs should be*)
Nice to know you. Not many guys from over there come in here.
Did you two walk all the way here? I mean, did you come all the
way from the front? That's a long way to --

                           BIG AL
It's okay. We took a short cut. Actually, we <u>made</u> us a short cut
through a hole in the fence.

                          JEREMY
It's really not that far. We're glad we found this place.

                            EVA
                    (*tapping BIG AL's patient
                     ID bracelet*)
Let's see, Shoff. You wearing one of these, too?

                          JEREMY
Yeah.

                            EVA
                    (*getting up to go back to
                     her bar stool*)
You two enjoy yourselves. Come in anytime and bring your friends
if you want. This is my bar and it's open to you anytime.

              *BAR PATRON brings over
              another pitcher of beer.*

                          JEREMY
I think we should call the others, Big Al. How about you?

                           BIG AL
                    (*looking at EVA*)
Yeah. I think that's a <u>really</u> good idea.

                          JEREMY
                    (*to Eva*)
Thanks, Eva, for that gracious invitation, and thanks, everyone,
for the beer! Would you keep Big Al company for a few minutes,
Eva? I'm going to call a few of our friends and tell them about
this great place we've found.

              *JEREMY walks behind the
              screen and you can hear
              his voice offstage.*

                    JEREMY (O.S.)
Hey, Earl Ray! We found a place just around the corner. Just
turn north when you come out the side doors. The Rainbow Bar and
Grille. Nice lady over here. Ya'll come quick. It's nice.
Real nice.
          (*walking back to the table*)
Any minute now. They'll be here any minute.

                    JEREMY and BIG AL drink
                    beer until EARL RAY, MOOSE,
                    BOBBY MAC and SKI come out
                    from behind the screen.

                    BIG AL
What took you so long?

                    JEREMY
Yeah. We got tired of waiting. Where's Pappy?

                    MOOSE
He's parking the car. If Earl doesn't like it here, he's ready
to take him back.

                    PAPPY comes in and sits
                    with them.

                    BIG AL
That was quick!

                    PAPPY
I sure don't want to miss out on a good thing.

                    EVA
Good to see you men. Let's see if we can fix you guys up.

                    EVA and BAR PATRON help
                    move the two tables stage
                    right and center together
                    and move the empty stools
                    to those tables, making
                    seven stools at the joined
                    tables and only two stools
                    at the table stage left.
                    EVA sits at the table stage
                    left and nods to BAR PATRON.

                    BAR PATRON
Looks like you men need another pitcher.

                    BAR PATRON carries over
                    another pitcher and five
                    more glasses, then joins
                    EVA at their table.

II-2-64

EARL RAY
The Rainbow. That's a hell-of-a-name for a bar.

BIG AL
Like I told Shoff, they could call it Hell for all I care. It's real close to the hospital, they got cold beer, and Eva is my kind of woman.

EARL RAY
Any woman is your kind of woman.

BIG AL
Not the kind of woman you're thinking of. She gives a shit.

EARL RAY
Ain't no woman gives a shit.

BIG AL
Why don't you find out for yourself?

EARL RAY
Yeah, right. Like some broad you met at a bar is going to give a shit about me.

BIG AL
She ain't some broad. If you got out once in a while, you'd see they ain't all broads.

EARL RAY
Why did she take a liking to your ass? It ain't like you got one.

BIG AL
She's just that way. Ain't that right, Shoff?

JEREMY
First woman I've ever known that gives a shit. She's real, Earl. She owns the place. Came right over to us and sat down next to Big Al.

BIG AL
She's a good dancer, too.

SKI
Her dname is Eva and she dances, too?

BIG AL
That's right, smart ass. And she bought us each a pitcher of beer.

EARL RAY
Remember. If I don't like it here, we ain't staying. Got it?

78

                              MOOSE
Got it, Earl.

                              BIG AL
Can we get four pitchers down here real quick?

                              EVA
No time to even say hello? What's the hurry? And why wouldn't
you like it here? Did these two tell you what a witch I am? The
name's Eva. And you are?

                              EARL RAY
Earl Ray.

                              EVA
Well, Earl Ray, you have a handsome face and wonderful blue eyes.
And your names?

               Each patient in turn says
               his name out loud.

                              EVA
Nice to meet all of you. I'll be back to check on you in a bit.

               EVA returns to the stage
               left table and nods at BAR
               PATRON to deliver four
               more pitchers of beer.

                              BIG AL
I told you she gives a shit.

                              EARL RAY
We've been here two minutes.

                              BIG AL
That's all you need.

                              MOOSE
What do you think, Earl? You want to stay awhile?

                              EARL RAY (*shrugging*)
Got nothing else to do.

                              JEREMY
Anybody need anything?

                              EARL RAY
Yeah. I want to see if that broad dances as good as Big Al says
she does.

                              BIG AL
She ain't a broad, Earl.

                        MOOSE
Okay, okay. Shoff, go see if she can settle this, will you?

            JEREMY walks over to EVA.

                        EVA
What's up, Shoff?

                        JEREMY
Earl Ray swears you can't dance.

                        EVA
Is that so? Seems Earl Ray needs a little personal attention.
Does he have any particular song in mind? Or is it my choice?

                        JEREMY
I think he would be glad if you did the honors.

            EVA moves behind the screen.

                        BIG AL
You must have scared the little lady.

                        EARL RAY
I knew she didn't give a shit.

                        BIG AL
Yeah, we'll see.

                        JEREMY
I think I could spend a lot of time here.

                        BOBBY MAC
You got that right. Shit, it may be just a little too close.
Look there, Shoff.

                        *EVA, who has added a slinky
                        dress over her hotpants,
                        dances gracefully from
                        behind the screen to EARL
                        RAY, never taking her eyes
                        off him.*

                        EVA
Just you and me, Earl.
            (*gently kissing EARL RAY*)
Just you and me.
            (*caressing EARL RAY's face*)
You are the bravest man I have ever met.

                        BIG AL
I told you so!

*Lights fade and go out,
one at a time, stage right
to stage left.*

ACT II

SCENE 3

SETTING: Rosie's Place. Stage right: two wheelchairs with a small table behind them. Stage left: two padded purple and lavender chairs with a matching couch, a coffee table, and a lamp with a fringed shade between them. A stand for the script is beside each chair, and another is beside the couch. An image of a purple curtain is projected on the screen.

AT RISE: As the lights come up on each seat in order from stage right to stage left, JEREMY and BIG AL are sitting in the wheelchairs stage right. ROSIE, smoking a cigarette and wearing a skirt split up the middle all the way up to her crotch, is watching them from one of the chairs stage left.

JEREMY
Man, I can't believe Pappy was deployed back to his duty station in Florida when he only had five months left. How're we ever going to get Earl Ray out of the hospital again?

BIG AL
I don't know. And just about the time I thought you and Pappy would finally prove Earl Ray wrong.

JEREMY
You mean about who we are? Well, you might have thought he'd change his mind about our being noncombat motherfuckers, but I don't think he ever will. Pappy and I will be noncombat motherfuckers to Earl till the day we die. Pass me that pack, will you?

BIG AL
(passing JEREMY a pack of
cigarettes)
It would have helped if he could have sold Earl that old Buick.

JEREMY
Yeah. That would have helped us get Earl back and forth to the Rainbow, for sure, but it was Pappy's only way to get back to his duty station in Florida. That car is all he had.

JEREMY
Well, until he gets out. He might come back. Five months, he said.

                              BIG AL
Who knows? Maybe he'll come back after that.

                    *JEREMY pulls two cigarettes
                    from the pack, lights them,
                    smokes one and hands the
                    other one to BIG AL.*

                              BIG AL
Thanks, my friend.

                    *ROSIE gets up out of her
                    chair and approaches BIG
                    AL and JEREMY.*

                              ROSIE
You two going to sit here all day?

                              BIG AL
Not me. It's hurting my ass.

                              ROSIE
The name's Rosie, nice to meet you two.

                              BIG AL
I'm Big Al, this here's Shoff.

                              ROSIE
Well, Big Al and Shoff, what brings you to my bus stop? My friends
and I have been watching you for almost half an hour.

                              BIG AL
Just resting a while. This walking takes a lot out of me.

                              ROSIE
I'm sure it does. Why don't you two come in and have a beer?

                              JEREMY/BIG AL
Are you kidding me? Sure!

                    *ROSIE and JEREMY, with
                    BIG AL around his neck,
                    cross the stage to her
                    living room.*

                              ROSIE
You two make yourselves comfortable. I'll get us something to
drink.

                    *ROSIE goes behind the
                    screen while BIG AL and
                    JEREMY sit and look around.*

JEREMY
(*excited and nervous*)
You thinking what I'm thinking?

BIG AL
(*excited*)
Yeah, Rosie runs a whore house! Somebody pinch me.

JEREMY
Of all the bus benches we could have picked. Damn good thing my legs were getting tired when they did.

BIG AL
Don't you dare take all the credit. Shit, it was my idea to give you a rest. I don't think we have enough money for this place.

JEREMY
That's for damn sure.

> *ROSIE comes back in with two mugs of beer and three glasses of wine on a tray.*

BIG AL
Wow, you really like your wine. And only one beer for us?

ROSIE
These are for my friends upstairs. Hope you like Budweiser.
(*laughing, Rosie puts the beer and one glass of wine on the table, then takes the other two wines offstage*)

JEREMY (*grinning*)
Did you hear that, Big Al? She has two friends upstairs!

BIG AL
(*tips his beer towards JEREMY*)
The King of Beers.

> *As ROSIE comes back in, BIG AL squirms on his chair.*

ROSIE
Would you be more comfortable sitting here, Al?

BIG AL
I'm okay. I'm just not used to nice pillows. The ones we have on Q are like bricks.

ROSIE
What's Q?

BIG AL
Oh, sorry. It's the ward we live on at the Navy hospital. Q ward.

ROSIE
(*raising her glass to toast*)
Well, here's to Q ward. And, I prefer to call this a Garden of Eden. Don't let Tammie and Sheryl hear you call it a whore house.

BIG AL
Sorry, we didn't mean anything by it. But you do -- you are -- I mean --

ROSIE
Yes, we do, and yes, we are. But we are very much ladies. And we don't walk the streets or hustle the bars.

JEREMY
Then how do you, you know.

ROSIE
We refer to them as clients, and they know how to find us. But this time we found you. Now, how do we get you upstairs, Big Al?

JEREMY
That's my job.

BIG AL
Can you believe this?
(*JEREMY carries BIG AL behind the screen and returns to the couch without him.*)

ROSIE
What about you, um, Shoff? Would you like to meet Sheryl?

JEREMY
I think I'll just wait for Big Al. You know we don't have a lot of mon --

ROSIE
Please, don't. You and your friend are our guests. We invited you here. We are doing this because we want to. Sure you don't want to meet Sheryl?

JEREMY
(*sitting on the couch*)
I'll just wait for Big Al.

ROSIE
(*sits next to JEREMY on the couch*)
She'll be more than disappointed. Are you trying to be noble?

JEREMY
No. I don't think I even know how to be. I just want this to be something special for Big Al.

ROSIE
What would Al say about you saying no?

JEREMY
He's going to think I'm nuts. He'll recommend me for the psych ward.

ROSIE
You can still change your mind.

JEREMY
Maybe next time. I mean if --

ROSIE
Of course, there will be a next time. You and Al are welcome anytime. Well, almost any time. We'll have to set up some rules. Let me think about it. I really don't like calling you Shoff. Do you have a first name?

JEREMY
Jeremy.

ROSIE
Well, Jeremy, what brought you two to my front gate.

JEREMY
Well, the Rainbow isn't the same without Earl Ray, so we were looking for a new place.

ROSIE
The Rainbow?

JEREMY
Yeah, the Rainbow. It's a bar close to the hospital.

ROSIE
And Earl Ray?

JEREMY
A friend of mine and Big Al's. A best friend.

ROSIE
He must be if you don't want to go to the Rainbow without him.

JEREMY
It's the only way we can get him out of the hospital. He lost both of his legs and his left arm in Viet Nam. The Rainbow is a special place for Earl Ray. It's where he can sit and talk with Eva. Sometimes they sit and talk for a couple of hours.

ROSIE

Who is Eva?

JEREMY

She owns the Rainbow. She's the only woman Earl Ray will talk to, well, except for Jennifer. And now, he doesn't talk to her very often.

ROSIE

Who's Jennifer?

JEREMY

Earl Ray's fiancé. She sends him letters every week. He just puts them in his locker unopened. Must be thirty or forty of them.

ROSIE

Why can't you get Earl Ray back over to the Rainbow?

JEREMY

Well, it's a long story. But mostly because Pappy left with his Buick and without his legs, Earl Ray doesn't have a way to get around.

ROSIE

I know that must make sense to you, Jeremy. But who's Pappy and what happened to him?

JEREMY

Pappy was another patient on Q. His ancient Buick was the only way to get Earl Ray over to the Rainbow. But then Pappy was sent back to full duty and Earl Ray hasn't left Q ward ever since.

ROSIE

It sounds like Earl Ray could use some personal attention. Maybe you can bring him by. Or maybe one of us could pick you guys up sometime. We'll talk about it.

JEREMY

That would be great if we could get him to come.

BIG AL (O.S.)
(*singing*)
Oh, Jeremy! I'm do-one! Come get me!

JEREMY goes behind the screen and comes back with BIG AL, who he helps into one of the chairs.

BIG AL

Oh, Jeremy! I think I'm in love! Tammie was magic.

                    ROSIE
You should see your cheeks, Al. Now you know why it's called
Rosie's Place.
          (to JEREMY)
See what you missed, Jeremy?

                    JEREMY
Man, I'm going to recommend myself to the psych ward.

                    BIG AL
What do mean? Didn't you? You what?

                    ROSIE
That's right, Al. He didn't.

                    BIG AL
You gotta be shitting me!

                    ROSIE
It's okay, Jeremy. Maybe next time? Speaking of next time. I've
thought about the rules. This is our secret; you tell anyone
other than Earl Ray and it's off. No more than once a week. After
all, it is a business. Call the number I gave you before you
want to come down. Friday and Sunday afternoons are best. Sit
on the bus bench until one of us comes out. Oh, and don't forget
to talk to Earl Ray.
          (kissing BIG AL and JEREMY
           on their cheeks)
And remember, we are ladies here.

                    JEREMY/BIG AL
Wow! Thank you, Rosie! Thanks for everything!

          JEREMY carries BIG AL
          back to the bench and sits
          next to him. They light
          cigarettes and smoke.

                    BIG AL
I think I'm in love, Shoff.

                    JEREMY
I don't blame you, Al.

                    BIG AL
No, I mean it. I think I'm in love. I could feel it. She held
me like a baby. I mean, she didn't just screw me, she made love
to me. I don't think I've ever had a woman do that before.

                    JEREMY
Be careful, Al, that's what she does for a living. Tammie may
not even be her real name.

BIG AL
I don't give a shit. I've never felt like that with a woman before.

JEREMY
Maybe it's the kind of women you've been with before.

BIG AL
She's different, man. I know she's supposed to make you feel good, but I'll bet other guys don't feel like this about her. Shit, they all probably got wives at home.

JEREMY
Let's talk about it back on Q.

BIG AL
No, I just want to sit here a while.

JEREMY
Okay with me. We've got all night.

JEREMY and BIG AL sit in silence for a moment.

BIG AL
I don't want to go back to Q.

JEREMY
We got to go in some time. People are going to wonder about us after a while.

BIG AL
No, Shoff, I really don't want to go back inside there.

JEREMY
Okay, Al. Whatever you want. We can sit here the rest of our lives if you want to.

BIG AL
I wish she hadn't been so nice to me. Ain't no way I'm going to meet another woman that can make me feel like she did.

JEREMY
I think there's women out there, Al. It just takes what it took tonight to find them.

BIG AL
Yeah, what's that?

JEREMY
Pure fucking luck.

                        BIG AL
Yeah, maybe you're right. Maybe it is pure fucking luck.
                    (*pause*)
C'mon, Shoff. Get me inside. I gotta piss.

        JEREMY laughs.

            The lights fade out, one
            at a time, stage right to
            stage left.

ACT II

SCENE 4

SETTING: *Rosie's Place. Stage right: two wheelchairs with a small table behind them. On the table is a rotary dial phone. Stage left: two padded purple and lavender chairs with a matching couch. Between them is a coffee table with a rotary dial phone on it and a lamp with a fringed shade. A stand for the script is beside each chair, and another is beside the couch. An image of a purple curtain is projected on the screen.*

AT RISE: *As the lights come up on each seat in order from stage right to stage left, JEREMY and BIG AL are sitting in the wheelchairs stage right. ROSIE, wearing a skirt split up the middle all the way up to her crotch, is sitting in one of the purple chairs.*

JEREMY walks to the rear of the stage, picks up the Q Ward phone and dials a number from a piece of paper. ROSIE answers.

ROSIE
(*into phone*)
Hello. This is Rosie.

JEREMY
(*into phone*)
Hi Rosie, it's Shoff.

ROSIE
(*into phone*)
Hi Jeremy. How have you been? I thought I would have heard from you sooner than this. Have you and Al forgotten about me?

JEREMY
(*into phone*)
Not hardly, Rosie. We've talked about you, Tammie, and Sheryl every day. Just me and Big Al that is. Well, and Earl Ray.

ROSIE
(*into phone*)
And what does Earl Ray think?

JEREMY
(*into phone*)
Just like Earl. At first, he said it was bullshit. The more we told him about it, the more he's convinced Big Al had a religious experience.

ROSIE
(*into phone*)
That's too funny.

JEREMY
(*into phone*)
Not for Big Al. He thinks he's in love with Tammie. He thinks if he stays away, he can forget about her.

ROSIE
(*into phone*)
And what do you think, Jeremy?

JEREMY
(*into phone*)
What do I think? Well, I think in his mind, he is in love with Tammie.

ROSIE
(*into phone*)
And does that bother you?

JEREMY
(*into phone*)
What would bother me is if Big Al gets screwed. I mean screwed over.

ROSIE
(*into phone*)
Trust me. Tammie knows what she's doing. She wants to see Al again.

JEREMY
(*into phone*)
Hold on a second. I want you to tell him what you just told me.

JEREMY carries BIG Al the phone.

BIG AL
(*into phone*)
Rosie? Big Al. How's it hangin'?

                    ROSIE
          (*into phone*)
Just fine, Al. Listen, this is a pretty good time for us. Why
don't you and Jeremy come on over? Tammie wants to see you.

          *BIG AL turns 360 degrees
          in his wheelchair.*

                    BIG AL
Shoff, I told you so!

                    JEREMY
          (*into phone*)
Rosie?

                    ROSIE
          (*into phone*)
Come on over, okay?

                    JEREMY
          (*into phone*)
We're on our way.

          *JEREMY picks up BIG AL
          and carries him across the
          stage, through ROSIE's
          living room, to behind the
          screen. ROSIE follows
          them. When they come back
          out, JEREMY is carrying
          BIG AL on his back, but is
          wearing only his uniform
          trousers and a tee shirt.
          ROSIE is carrying JEREMY's
          uniform shirt. JEREMY
          puts BIG AL in one of the
          chairs, and JEREMY and
          ROSIE sit on the couch.*

                    ROSIE
That was nice. We'll have to do this again sometime.

                    JEREMY
That would be nice, Rosie.

                    ROSIE
You two look ecstatic. Would you like something to drink?

                    JEREMY
A couple of beers would be great. Thanks, Rosie.

                    ROSIE
Nice to see everyone smiling. Must have been a good afternoon.

II-4-80

JEREMY
The only thing better would have been Earl Ray with us.

BIG AL
Yeah. If we could only get him here.

ROSIE
I've heard a lot about Earl Ray. When do you think I can meet him?

JEREMY
We're not sure Earl Ray wants to go anywhere. Sometimes he thinks he's a pain in the ass to everybody, including himself.

BIG AL
Shit, we'd take him anywhere he wants. We'd do anything for him. He just doesn't see it that way. Besides, I think it's mostly Jennifer.

ROSIE
From what you've told me, Jeremy, Jennifer's his whole life. Or used to be. Tell you what. If you can get Earl Ray to say yes to me, I'm sure Sheryl would be more than happy to come pick him up.

BIG AL
It's worth a try. He needs to get out before he goes nuts or drives us nuts.

JEREMY
He needs to get out before he does something we'll all regret.

ROSIE
What do you mean by that, Jeremy?

JEREMY
We promised him he could choose to end his life. If that's what he wants. We promised we wouldn't stop him.

ROSIE
Then let's get him over here and see if we can convince him he doesn't want to do that.

*Lights fade and go out,
one at a time, stage right
to stage left.*

ACT II

SCENE 5

SETTING: *Rosie's Place. Stage right: two wheelchairs with a small table behind them. Stage left: two padded purple and lavender chairs with a matching couch, and a lamp with a fringed shade on a coffee table between them. A stand for the script is beside each chair and another is beside the couch. An image of a purple curtain is projected on the screen.*

AT RISE: *As the lights come up on each seat in order from stage right to stage left, JEREMY, carrying BIG AL on his back and pushing EARL RAY's wheelchair, follows ROSIE into her living room. EARL RAY is carrying crutches. ROSIE is wearing a skirt split up the middle all the way up to her crotch. With BIG AL still on his back, JEREMY parks EARL RAY's chair next to Rosie's.*

ROSIE
Tammie is waiting and time is wasting, don't you think, Al?

BIG AL
We'll see you guys in a couple of hours. Don't do anything I wouldn't do!

JEREMY carries BIG AL behind the screen.

ROSIE
We're so glad you decided to come, Earl. We've heard a lot about you. You have two very special friends.

EARL RAY
Big Al, maybe. I'm not sure I would call Shoff special.

JEREMY comes back out and sits on the couch.

JEREMY
You'll never get a Marine to call anyone in the Navy special.

EARL RAY
Got that right, noncombat -- I won't say that in front of the ladies.

ROSIE
Thank you, Earl for calling us ladies. We love you already.

ROSIE
What about you, Earl? Sheryl would like to get to know you.
(*pointing towards screen*)
If you'd like to get to meet her, she's right through there.

EARL RAY
I don't know. Maybe some other time.

ROSIE
It's okay. You can just talk if you want. She won't do anything you don't want to do.

EARL RAY
Okay. I'll give it a try. Just get me in there, Shoff, then get out.

JEREMY pushes EARL RAY behind the beaded screen, with ROSIE following.

EARL RAY (O.S.)
Give me my crutches, Shoff! I can do this myself!

JEREMY (O.S.)
Get one under his right arm, Rosie!

ROSIE (O.S.)
Got it, Jeremy. You're okay, Earl.

EARL RAY (O.S.)
I'm okay. Just wasn't watching where I was going. Now, get out of here, Shoff! I don't need your fucking help!

ROSIE and JEREMY return to the living room and sit on the couch.

EARL RAY (O.S.)
Told you, Shoff!

JEREMY
I never doubted it, Earl.

ROSIE
He means a lot to you, doesn't he, Jeremy?

JEREMY
He's my hero, Rosie. And you know what? He's never asked for a fucking thing. Not one god damn thing. He's more of a man than I'll ever be. And don't dare pity him.
(MORE)

                        JEREMY (CONT'D)
He'll kill you if you do. Don't let him see you give a shit,
either. No, don't do that. That means he has to give a shit
back. That's the way he is. There's only so much loyalty for
him to give, but when he does give it to you, it matters. It
means something. Ask Ski and Moose and Big Al. Ask any Marine.
Ask Jennifer. I'll never earn it. I've tried. I don't deserve
it. He tried to kill me once. He could have, too, but I believe
he really didn't want to. He's accepted me, but he'll never trust
me. He pushes back on every fucking thing. He pisses me off,
but I think he knows I love him like a brother. He deserves more
than any of us can ever give him, but he'll never take anything
from anyone he doesn't trust. Don't ever owe anybody anything.
That's Earl -- and he's never once asked for a god damn thing.

                            ROSIE
C'mon Jeremy, let's go upstairs.

                    *JEREMY and ROSIE go hand-
                    in-hand behind the screen.*

                            FEMALE VOICE (O.S.)
Help me! Someone help! Please hurry!

                            JEREMY (O.S.)
Holy shit! He's having a flashback! He might be killing her!

                            BIG AL (O.S.)
Get me in there, Shoff! Quick! Hurry, Shoff!

                            JEREMY (O.S.)
We're coming, Earl. Hold on, Earl. Just hold on.

                            FEMALE VOICE (O.S.)
I'm okay. Really. It's just that my pubic hairs are stuck in
his legs. Please help me get them out. As fast as you can.

                            BIG AL (O.S.)
Oh, wow! Just hold really still, okay Earl? We can fix this.

                            EARL RAY (O.S.)
Get me out of here. Get me back to Q.

                            FEMALE VOICE (O.S.)
It's okay, Earl. What if we take them off? I'll be okay, I think.

                            EARL RAY (O.S.)
Just get me out of here and get me back to Q.

                            ROSIE (O.S.)
Maybe we can sit in the living room for a while.

                            JEREMY (O.S.)
What do you think, Al?

                    BIG AL (O.S.)
    Just get me back to Q, Shoff. Get us back to Q.

                    Lights fade out and turn
                    off, one at a time, stage
                    right to stage left.

ACT II

SCENE 6

BIG AL

SETTING: *The Bus. Seven wheelchairs are in a row, each facing stage left. The one in front (for the "bus driver") has a space between it and the others. The image of a Navy bus is projected on the screen. A stand for the script is beside each chair.*

AT RISE: *As the lights come up on each seat in order from stage right to stage left, the back wheelchair is empty. SKI, BOBBY MAC, MOOSE, BIG AL, and EARL RAY are sitting in the wheelchairs facing stage left. TINY, in his Navy corpsman first class uniform, and JEREMY, in his Navy everyday whites, are standing beside "the bus". The Marines are all in their non-dress, khaki uniforms.*

TINY
(*shaking Jeremy's hand*)
Jeremy, it's been my pleasure to have you work for me in Special Services these past few months. Today's trip is the last one of the summer, and, as you know, it is indeed special.

JEREMY
Thanks, Tiny. It's been fun, and you helped make it that way. I think I can speak for everybody here, this trip to Atlantic City for the weekend is something we all thank you for. We know how lucky we are to have been picked for this trip.

TINY
You're lucky <u>any</u> of you were <u>ever</u> picked for another trip after that last clam bake!

JEREMY
Well, if the band hadn't played "Mr. Lonely" and dedicated "Coming Home Soldier" to -- and I quote -- "their special audience," all of those emotions wouldn't have swept through the festivities like a fire through a funeral pyre. But, oh, my God, wasn't it a great ending to the day? Corn cobs, chicken bones, clam shells, and paper plates flying everywhere? Tables and wheelchairs and plastic and wooden body parts all over the place, and people hiding under the tables and tablecloths? God, it was <u>great</u>. I think the only thing not being thrown was the beer, and that's only because we were drinking it as fast as we could.

                    TINY (*laughing*)
Okay, well, that was pretty spectacular. And then for it to stop,
all of a sudden, with everyone laughing, shaking hands, and
embracing? It was, I admit, one of the coolest things I've ever
seen. And just so you know, when I asked "What are you going to
do for an encore," that didn't mean you should repeat the
performance this weekend.

                    JEREMY
Wouldn't think of it, Tiny. We'll be on our best behavior. I
promise.

                    *JEREMY and TINY enter
                    "the bus," TINY standing
                    at the front, facing the
                    wheelchairs, and JEREMY
                    going to the back.*

                    TINY
So, who's gonna win?
                    (*confused looks from the
                    others*)
Miss America, you bums! That's why we're going to Atlantic City
for crying out loud.

                    JEREMY/SKI/MOOSE
Oh!

                    MOOSE
I don't even know who's in the contest.

                    TINY
For God's sake. Just name a state!

                    EARL RAY
Shit, Moose, you ever hear of Miss America before today?

                    BOBBY MAC
You got fifty chances. Go for it.

                    BIG AL
I don't care who wins. Ain't none of them can come close to Tammie.

                    EARL RAY
I still don't know why she's taken a liking to your ass.

                    BIG AL
What's it matter, Earl? She's a lot like Jennifer, you know.

                    EARL RAY
What do you know about it?

                        BIG AL
I know Jennifer would give her life for you. Shit, man. Wake up
before it's too late.

                        EARL RAY
                (*raising his prosthetic arm
                and hook into the air*)
Look at me. It's already too late.

                        SKI
Eets never too late. Dyou should read Jendeefer's letters. How
the hell dyou know if eets too late.

                        EARL RAY
'Cause I said so. Maybe I don't want to know what is in those
letters.

                        BOBBY MAC
You keep them for a reason, my friend.

                        EARL RAY
                (*staring out the window*)
Well, it's none of your business.

                        MOOSE
You're one of us, Earl. That makes it our business.

                        EARL RAY
                (*reaching in shirt pocket*)
The only thing that would help right now is another pain pill,
and for you guys to shut up about it.

                        MOOSE
Okay, Earl. We'll give it a break for now. Just be careful with
those things. You scared the shit out of us the last time you
took too many.

                        EARL RAY
You can never take too many.

                        BOBBY MAC
Got to take it easy with that shit, Earl. We need you around to
keep us in line. We all need some of it, but take it easy.

                        EARL RAY
Just back off for now.

                        TINY
                (*putting a hand on EARL
                RAY's shoulder*)
They're right, Earl. You and I have talked about this before. I
should have reported it the last time, but God help me, I didn't.
I can't keep turning a blind eye.

                              EARL RAY
I'm okay, Tiny. I'm okay.

                              TINY
We better get going. It's four hours to the hotel and they have a Friday night all-you-can-eat buffet waiting for us.

                              SKI
WoooHooo! Follow dthe yellow brick droad!

> *TINY and JEREMY sit in their seats. A female HIPPIE wearing hippie clothes and SGT. PEPPER, a long-haired male in his early twenties wearing Marine corps fatigues, both adorned with peace emblem headbands, hippie hats and leather fringe vests, enter the stage from stage left and step in front of the bus.*

                              HIPPIE
                     (*flipping them the finger*)
Hey, fuck you, baby killers!

                              SGT. PEPPER
I'm ashamed of what I did in Nam, and you should be, too!

                              MOOSE
Fuck you, you long-haired motherfucker! Stay right there and I'll baby-kill your ass!

                              BOBBY MAC
Yeah, you chicken-shit asshole!

                              SGT. PEPPER
                     (*giving the finger*)
Fuck you, man! You baby-killing bastards!

> *As HIPPIE stands in front of bus, SGT. PEPPER moves to beside EARL RAY.*

                              EARL RAY
                     (*hitting in SGT. PEPPER's direction*)
How 'bout this, motherfucker!

                              SGT. PEPPER
Shit! What the fuck! I'll kill <u>your</u> ass.

                           TINY
               (*TINY, MOOSE and JEREMY
                jump off the bus and start
                pounding on SGT. PEPPER.*)
Okay, asshole. Who's next?

                          HIPPIE
Get off him! Get off him!

                           TINY
               (*grabbing MOOSE's shoulder*)
Okay, Moose. He's had enough. Jeremy, get off of him.

                         JEREMY
               (*punching SGT. PEPPER one
                more time*)
You don't ever talk to my friends like that! You got it!

                           TINY
Now, you assholes get away from my bus!

               *HIPPIE helps SGT. PEPPER
               move to behind the bus.*

                          HIPPIE
We didn't know, man. I mean -- we thought --.

                           TINY
You take another step and I'll put your ass on that bus! That what you want?

                        BOBBY MAC
               (*through the window*)
C'mon, you long-haired assholes! Get on the bus. We'll give you a ride you won't forget!

                           SKI
Open dthe door! Don't dcall me a babykeeler, you modorfowkers!

                         EARL RAY
Get over here! I'll gouge your fucking eyes out!

                      TINY (*shouting*)
I said get the fuck out of here!

                       SGT. PEPPER
We're sssssorry, man. We didn't mmmmean no harm. We're sssssorry, man. We didn't mmmmean no harm.

                           TINY
Well, we did! Now get the hell out of my sight!

                    TINY, MOOSE and JEREMY
                    get back on the bus to
                    cheering from everyone
                    else. As TINY takes his
                    seat, he smiles broadly.

                              TINY
This is going to be an <u>exceptional</u> trip.

                    Lights fade and go out,
                    one at a time, stage right
                    to stage left.

ACT II

SCENE 7

SETTING: Atlantic City. Six stools and two wheelchairs are arranged around two bar-height (for the stools) and one lower (for the wheelchairs) tables. After the lights come up, an image of a high-class hotel lounge is projected on the screen. A stand for the script is on each table.

AT RISE: BOBBY MAC, MOOSE, SKI, JEREMY and TINY are sitting on the stools. EARL RAY and BIG AL are sitting in the wheelchairs. TINY is in his Navy corpsman first class uniform, JEREMY is in his Navy everyday whites, and the Marines are all in their non-dress, khaki uniforms. ESCORT and DAVE are standing to one side.

In the dark, before the lights come up, an ANNOUNCER's booming voice is heard.

MALE VOICE (O.S.)
Ladies and gentlemen. It is my great pleasure and honor to welcome our special guests this evening. Please join me in giving a big round of applause for the group of Vietnam Veterans from the U.-S. Naval Hospital in Philadelphia! We are thankful for their service and their individual sacrifices. Welcome, veterans, to the Miss America Pageant, and thank you!

All cast members applaud.

Lights come up, one at a time, stage right to stage left. The patients and Tiny are all sitting around the tables.

EARL RAY
What the fuck kind of name is Reg Morgan for a bar?

BIG AL
Hey, the guy at the pageant said this is a great place. It's gotta be better than that beauty contest. Anyway, they can call it Hell for all I care. Just get me a beer.

                    DAVE
          (*coming to their table and
           sitting on the empty stool*)
Hey, ain't you guys the veterans that were at the beauty pageant
tonight? The ones in the spotlights?

                    MOOSE
Yeah, that's us.

                    DAVE
You guys are the ones who've been to Vietnam? You're over in
Philly, right?

                    MOOSE
Yeah, that's us. You're not looking for trouble are you?

                    DAVE
Hell no. This is your lucky night. The name's Dave Marzetti. I
own this bar. Tonight, you guys help yourselves. Tonight, the
bar's all yours. And you ain't going to pay a dime. Just ask
for whatever you want. What'll you have?

                    SKI
Scotch and soda.

                    DAVE
What the hell. You don't need someone to mix your drinks for
you. You guys can just mix your own. You don't need anyone else
to do this. All you need is the booze.
          (*waves at ESCORT, who brings
           over glasses and bottles
           of gin, vodka, whiskey and
           scotch along with mixers*)

                    DAVE
You guys got everything you need? Anything you want, just ask
for it. I'll get someone to get it for you.

                    SKI
          (*with a sly grin*)
Well, dwe could always use a woman or two.

                    DAVE
          (*smiling and putting his
           arm around Ski*)
I should have known. Just give me a minute.
          (*walks behind the screen*)

                    BIG AL
Who's the scary looking guy following Dave around?

                    BOBBY MAC
It's Dave's bodyguard, would be my guess.

BIG AL
What does he need a bodyguard for?

BOBBY MAC
Because he does shit other people don't like, that's why.

BIG AL
What kinda things?

MOOSE
What's it fuckin' matter? He's doin' right by us, isn't he?

BIG AL
Hell, yeah!

DAVE
(*has a word with ESCORT and then comes back to their table, bringing ESCORT with him*)
Come on you guys! We have a special room in the back for our special friends, if you know what I mean. My friend here is going to take each of you for a ride! And I mean a ride!

ESCORT
Come with me, gentlemen. Which of you handsome men wants to go first?

The patients and TINY all look at each other, then back to the ESCORT.

DAVE
What are you waiting for?

MOOSE
That's all the encouragement I need.

BOBBY MAC
Oh shit, we don't need privacy! I'm going to watch. Been so long I think I forgot how!

MOOSE and BOBBY MAC leave with ESCORT and follow her behind the screen.

EARL RAY
Just like the choppers in Nam, this is the jump seat. Even for you, Shoff.

JEREMY
(*holding up a drink*)
I'll drink to that!

                              BIG AL
Shoff, you're _my_ jump seat. Be ready when I am!

                              JEREMY
Alright, Big Al. This chopper's gonna fly.

                              DAVE
Next?

                              BIG AL
Get me in there, Shoff!

              JEREMY pushes BIG AL in
              his wheelchair behind the
              screen as MOOSE and BOBBY
              MAC come out smiling.

                              JEREMY
                    (*returning to his seat*)
How about you, Earl? You ready to jump?

                              EARL RAY
You go ahead, Shoff.

                              JEREMY
You go, Earl. I'll get my turn.

                              EARL RAY
                    (*looking at the floor*)
No, you go, Shoff. I don't think I can do it.

                              BOBBY MAC
Sure you can, Earl. Just lay down and let her do the rest!

                              EARL RAY
It's not that, man. It's Jennifer.

                              JEREMY
Okay, I'll jump next!

                              SKI
Don't forget dme. I weel go next!

                              TINY
Not me! I know they'll make anyone who takes a turn get tested
tomorrow.

                              EARL RAY
You better hope none of you bastards have the clap.

                              BIG AL
Too late now! I still got the fungus from Nam!

                    BOBBY MAC
If you still got that shit from Nam, your dick would've fallen
off by now!

          ESCORT comes back out,
          assisting BIG AL in his
          wheelchair.

                    BIG AL
Yeah, well go ask the blonde about my dick.

                    SKI
My deek better not fall off. I dwill keek what's left of your
ass!

          ESCORT leads JEREMY and
          SKI to the back room.

                    MOOSE
Everybody who wants one get at least one jump?

                    BIG AL
Two for me!

                    TINY
Hey guys, it's almost five in the morning. We better get back.

                    DAVE
How would you guys like a little breakfast? I know where there's
a great buffet.

                    TINY
Thanks, Dave, but we really need to get back as soon as Jeremy
and Ski come out. If we don't get back soon, they'll put us down
as AWOL.

                    DAVE
Okay, but I'm getting your cabs back to your hotel. Here's a
business card for each one of you. If you're ever in Atlantic
City, call me. And if you ever are here and <u>don't</u> call me, I'll
know.

          JEREMY and SKI come back
          out from behind the screen.

                    TINY
On behalf of all of us, thank you, Dave! It has been an
outstanding night!

                    DAVE
Any time, men. Any time. It's been an honor.

          All the men shake hands
          and say their goodbyes.

II-7-96

> *As they head towards the door, TINY points to MOOSE, BIG AL, SKI, BOBBY MAC, and JEREMY.*

TINY
You, you, you, you and you! All of you but Earl Ray are going with me down to sick bay tomorrow. That little episode has earned you a reward. You're all getting squeezed for V.-D.

JEREMY
What's he mean, squeezed?

BOBBY MAC
It ain't really squeezed, it's more like poked.

ROGER
The fickle finger of fate.

SKI
Dright up dthe old pooper.

MOOSE
No big deal! Just bend over and enjoy it.

> *They are all laughing and staggering as they go off the stage, with their arms around each other's shoulders.*
>
> *Lights fade and go out, one at a time, stage right to stage left.*

ACT II

SCENE 8

SETTING: *Q Ward. A photo of the hospital is projected onto a screen behind the actors. A full-length mirror stands beside the screen.*

In an arc across the stage from stage right to stage left are: three empty wheelchairs, a stool, a footlocker on which there is a bottle of Jack Daniels and a small box, EARL RAY in his wheelchair, wearing his full Marine Corps dress uniform with medals and ribbons, and two more empty wheelchairs. Two prosthetic legs and an arm hang on the side of EARL RAY's wheelchair. He is holding a bottle of pills and a pile of letters is in his lap. In front of each seat is a stand for the script.

AT RISE: *As the lights come up on each seat in order from stage right to stage left, JEREMY, MOOSE, BIG AL, BOBBY MAC, and SKI come in from stage right. JEREMY is in wearing his Navy everyday white uniform, All the Marines are wearing their non-dress, USMC khaki uniforms. They all go quiet and stare when they see EARL RAY.*

MOOSE

What's up, Earl?

EARL RAY

The sky.

MOOSE

You know what I mean. C'mon, what's going on?

EARL RAY

Just let it happen. Don't call for help until you're certain it's too late. Keep your promise. I'm feeling really lucky today.

MOOSE
 (*picking up the bottle of pills*)
How many did you take?

                          EARL RAY
Not enough.

                          MOOSE
How did you get so many, Earl? That's twice what they give you
at the pharmacy.

                          EARL RAY
Shit, Moose, I can get twenty of these for a pack of smokes.

                          MOOSE
How many did you take, my friend?

                          EARL RAY
Four -- maybe five. I'm not sure. Probably not enough.

                          MOOSE
Then let's call it quits for now. What do you say?

                          EARL RAY
Just let it happen this time. You guys promised.

                          MOOSE
Don't let this be the last thing you do with your life, Earl.

                          EARL RAY
It's not, Moose. The last thing I did with my life was step on a
land mine.

                          BIG AL
Jesus, Earl. Think about it for a while, huh?

                          EARL RAY
Shit, Al. You know damn well I've <u>been</u> thinking about it. I've
been thinking about it for a long <u>time</u>, for Christ's sake. Don't
stop me. Just stay close by. That's all I ask.

                          SKI
I dknow we promised, Earl. Eef eet's what dyou want weel be here.
But, I'm asking you to not to do eet.

                          JEREMY
                (*blurts out*)
I've changed my mind, Earl! I'm going for help.

                          EARL RAY
You can't, god dammit. You made a promise. All of you.

                          MOOSE
                (*picking up the bottle of
                 Jack*)
Let me have a drink of the Jack. Okay, Earl? Why don't you give
me the pills, too.

                    EARL RAY
Can't do it, Moose. Even if I don't do it now, I'll need these
when the time comes. But like I said, I'm feeling really lucky.

>   *A phone is heard ringing
>   repeatedly off-stage, then
>   stops. A few seconds later
>   a VOICE is heard yelling
>   from offstage.*

                    MALE VOICE (O.S.)
Some girl on the phone wants to talk to an Earl Ray. Says her
name is Jennifer. She's calling from the front gate.

                    JEREMY
You stay here and I'll bring you the phone, Earl. The cord is
long enough to reach in here.

>   *JEREMY goes behind the
>   screen and returns carrying
>   a rotary-dial phone, which
>   he holds as he hands the
>   handset to EARL RAY.*

                    EARL RAY
          (*into phone*)
Is this some kind of a fucking joke!
          (*pause*)
Who is this really?
          (*pause*)
Jen? Is it really you?
          (*pause*)
Jen. Jen, it's really you?
          (*pause*)
You're _where_? You're at the front gate _here_? At the hospital?
          (*pause*)
What are you doing here?
          (*pause*)
You want to take me home? Now? You're taking me _home_?
          (*weeping*)
Oh, Babe. Oh, Babe. Yes. I'll go with you. I'll get the guys
to help me and I'll be right down.
          (*Hangs up phone and hands
          it back to JEREMY. Looks
          up at MOOSE.*)
I'm going home, guys. I'm going home.

>   *All the patients cheer
>   loudly. They are laughing,
>   celebrating, and slapping
>   each other on the backs as
>   DR. DONNOLLY enters the
>   ward and slowly walks over
>   to them.*

                        BIG AL
Dr. Donnolly. What's wrong? What are you doing out here?

                        EARL RAY
You look terrible. It's no fucking good, is it?

                        DR. DONNOLLY
No it's not, Earl. I thought it would be best if you guys heard it from me.

                        BIG AL
What could be that bad?

                        DR. DONNOLLY (*choking up*)
I'm sorry to have to tell you this, but Doc Miller was killed in Viet Nam.

> *The patients stop, stunned, and look back and forth from DR. DONNOLLY to each other. No one speaks. All at once, the stage goes dark.*
>
> *PLEASE NOTE: This is the only scene in the entire play for which all the lights go out at the same time.*

ACT II

SCENE 9

SETTING: *The Rainbow Bar and Grille. Stage right: Two bar-height tables are placed together with six stools behind them. EVA and the BAR PATRON are sitting behind a third table at stage left. A photo of the interior of a neighborhood bar is projected on the screen behind the actors.*

AT RISE: *As the lights come up on each seat in order from stage right to stage left, JEREMY, MOOSE, BIG AL, BOBBY MAC, and SKI enter the Rainbow. JEREMY is carrying BIG AL, and is in wearing his Navy everyday white uniform, All the Marines are wearing their non-dress, USMC khaki uniforms. They sit at the tables.*

EVA
(walking over to the booth where the group is seated)
Hey guys. Where have you been for so long? Is my dancing that bad? And where's Earl Ray? I've missed him.

MOOSE
He's in Florida, soaking up some sun and some lovin'. Jennifer took him home. You should have seen him the day she pulled up to Q ward. First time we ever saw him smile. We miss him, too.

EVA
So what's the occasion for your coming back?

MOOSE
Shoff has news, and he wouldn't tell us till we got here.

BIG AL
Yeah. What's such a big deal you couldn't tell us on Q?

EVA
Let's hear it, Jeremy. You look like you're about to bust.

JEREMY
(grinning)
I couldn't be better!

BOBBY MAC
What are you so happy about? You getting out of here?

                    JEREMY
Yeah. I got my review board decision today.

                    SKI
Dyou are geeting out? Dyou are going home?

                    BOBBY MAC
Oh man, that's great!

                    JEREMY
No, guys, I ain't getting out. I got my orders, but they got me fit for full duty. Gave me orders for an aircraft carrier. I'm headed for Nam.

                    BIG AL
No way! They can't do that.

                    JEREMY
They've done it. That admiral I pissed off made sure the brass here didn't forget. He got the review board to overrule Dr. Donnolly. But it's no big deal. I owe you guys at least a trip over there.

                    BIG AL
You don't owe us shit. You serious? The boat you're goin' on is headed to Nam?

                    JEREMY
That's what they say.

                    BOBBY MAC
Now ain't that some shit.

                    JEREMY
You guys know it don't mean shit to be on a boat near Nam.

                    MOOSE
Well, I'll be a son of a bitch.

                    BIG AL
They got you, didn't they?

                    JEREMY
That's what it's all about. They made sure that smart-ass remark I made to the admiral stayed in my records. And my mother's phone call to her congressman didn't help much either.

                    SKI
dWhat phone call? dWhat Congressman?

JEREMY
It wasn't much. I happened to mention to my mom what the admiral had done and she wrote some congressman a letter. I got called down by the legal dudes to explain why I was trying to ruin the reputation of the hospital and the good doctors here. Something about a possible congressional inquiry, too. I signed a couple of forms and never heard shit after that.

BIG AL
Holy shit! Your ass is grass even on that boat!

JEREMY
They can fuck with me all they want. Don't mean shit.

MOOSE
Ain't no way you're gonna go. We'll talk to Dr. Donnolly.

JEREMY
He's already talked to the board. They don't give a shit what he says. I don't think they'll even put his report in my file.

SKI
Shit, man, dthey got us all by dthe balls if they want.

BOBBY MAC
You just finding that out? Be glad you still got balls!

MOOSE
Let me guess. You're telling us here because this calls for a party!

EVA
Got that right! And not just any old party. The Rainbow's gonna do it big and do it right tonight! The beer's on the house tonight. It'll be a party of which Earl Ray would be proud.

BIG AL
Sounds good to me! We need more beer.

> *EVA nods at BAR PATRON, who brings four more pitchers of beer.*

MOOSE
When you gotta report?

JEREMY
I got one week left here.

BOBBY MAC
Well ain't that some shit. Uncle Sam took a dump on Shoff and we're here to wash him off! We're gonna need a lot of beer to get rid of the stink.

                              EVA
Well, don't get any of it on my bar. What did you do, Jeremy, to
deserve this?

                              SKI
He peesed off the big brass over a dyear ago and they didn't forget
it.

                              EVA
Must have been serious if they held a grudge this long.

                              MOOSE
They don't forget shit. The higher-ups are protecting their own
asses.

                              EVA
What is it <u>exactly</u> that you did?

                              BIG AL
He told the admiral to shove it!

                              EVA
An admiral? That was a crazy thing to do, Jeremy.

                              MOOSE
Crazy enough we made him an honorary Marine!

                              BOBBY MAC
An honorary Marine and by-God relative, too! Let's fucking
celebrate!

                              JEREMY
                    (*lifting his beer*)
To Doc.

               *All present lift their
               glasses in a silent toast.*

                              EVA
Say, you guys got quiet all of a sudden. What happened?

                              MOOSE
We were just saluting one of the best corpsman in the Navy.

                              BIG AL
                    (*raising his glass of beer*)
No, to <u>the</u> best corpsman in the Navy.

                              BOBBY MAC
Yeah, here's to Doc Miller.

                              EVA
Well, why didn't you bring him with you? Where is he?

MOOSE
He's not here.

EVA
You mean he was transferred?

MOOSE
No. He's gone. Vietnam.

EVA
When is he coming home? Do you know?

MOOSE
He ain't coming home. He didn't make it.

EVA
(*crying and walking away*)
I am so sorry. When is all of this <u>ever</u> going to stop?

SKI
What do dyou say we call eet a night?

BIG AL
Yeah, we may as well head back.

BAR PATRON
How about another round for you guys, before you go?

BOBBY MAC
Thanks, man, but we're going to call it a night.

MOOSE
I've been thinking, Shoff. Like I've been saying, ain't no way you're going to get on that boat.

JEREMY
Says who?

MOOSE
Says me. They can't fuck with you like that, so you ain't going.

JEREMY
How am I going to get out of it? I ain't going to Canada.

BOBBY MAC
You're damn right, you're not.

JEREMY
Then what do you plan to do? Hide me on Q?

MOOSE
Nope. We're going to break your legs. You can't leave here with two broken legs.

JEREMY (*gulping*)
Break my legs?

MOOSE
That's right. Been thinking about this all evening, Shoff. It wouldn't take much. Just a table ought'a do it.

JEREMY
How the hell we going to explain it?

MOOSE
Shit, we'll just tell them we got in a bar fight.

SKI
I don't dknow about theese. Just geeve eet a break.

BOBBY MAC
Ain't this some shit! Let me help you with that, Moose! Wish to hell I had thought of it.

MOOSE
Okay, Shoff, all you'll have to do is sit down and put your legs straight out. We'll take care of the rest.

SKI
dYou are serious?

BOBBY MAC
Serious as a fucking bad land mine!

BIG AL
C'mon. Ain't no way we can let those bastards get away with it.

JEREMY
Damn right. Go for it, Moose.

MOOSE
What do you think, Ski?

SKI
Okay, if eet's okay with dyou, Jeremy.

JEREMY
What have I got to lose?

JEREMY stretches out his legs.

BOBBY MAC
You ready for this, Shoff?

SKI
An honorary dMarine is always ready!

BIG AL
Oh shit!

BOBBY MAC
On the count of three.

BIG AL
Oh, shit!

MOOSE
Ready?
(*lifting a table over his head*)
One!

BIG AL
Oh, shit!

MOOSE
Two!

BIG AL
Oh shit!

EVA
(*comes running over*)
What the hell are you guys doing? Good God, you need to stop that! Are you trying to kill him?

BOBBY MAC
Hell no, we're saving his life!

MOOSE drops the table.

MOOSE
Oh shit!

SKI
Sawnoffabeedtch! Look what dyou did dnow!

EVA
Good Grief! Stop all this craziness and just get back to the hospital! I'll call you a cab.

Lights fade and go out one at a time, stage right to stage left.

ACT II

SCENE 10

SETTING: Q Ward. A photo of Jeremy in his uniform is projected onto a screen behind the actors. A full-length mirror stands beside the screen.

In an arc across the stage from stage right are: BOBBY MAC, JEREMY, and SKI in their wheelchairs, a stool, a footlocker, an empty wheelchair where EARL RAY used to sit, and MOOSE and BIG AL in their wheelchairs. Two prosthetic legs and an arm hang on the side of EARL RAY's old wheelchair. In front of each seat is a stand for the script.

AT RISE: As the lights come up on each seat in order from stage right to stage left, JEREMY, in his full dress blues, stands and picks up his sea bag.

MOOSE
We can still do it, you know. It's not too late.

JEREMY
Yeah, but I'm sober now. Things look a little different than they did a week ago. Besides, it's a damn ship. It ain't like I'm going on a patrol boat.

MOOSE
(lifting his left arm stump)
Tell me about it.

SKI
Yeah, at least dthey didn't screw dyou like dthat.

BOBBY MAC
They're good at screwing everybody. One way or the other.

PAPPY, in his Coast Guard uniform, enters stage right.

MOOSE
Well, look here! Ain't this some shit! What the hell are you doing here?

BIG AL (*hopefully*)
Pappy? The limo is back?

PAPPY
I took an early out. Couldn't see driving all the way to Florida just to turn around and drive back here. I got two weeks until I'm discharged from the Coast Guard.

BOBBY MAC
Well, son of a bitch. Welcome back to Q, Pappy the Sailor! By God, welcome back!

BIG AL
(*rolls over to look outside*)
It's here! The most beautiful thing I've seen since Tammie.

PAPPY
I thought maybe I could make a beer run later on.

MOOSE
Better make it quick. Shoff here's just getting ready to leave us.

PAPPY
Where're you going, Shoff? You getting out?

JEREMY
No early out for me, Pappy. I have a flight in a couple of hours. Going to San Diego and then off to see the world.

MOOSE
He's on the brass' shit list big time. They're sending him to Nam on a carrier.

BOBBY MAC
Just make it back in one piece, you got that, Shoff?

JEREMY
How will guys you ever know? We'll probably never see each other again.

PAPPY
If you don't mind, Jeremy, it would be my pleasure to take you to the airport.

JEREMY
(*shaking hands with MOOSE
and BOBBY MAC*)
We better get going then. I don't want to hold up a beer run.

MOOSE
You're not too bad for a noncombat mother -- for an honorary Marine.

JEREMY (*laughing*)
Thank you, my friend. Thank you.

> *JEREMY reaches down and shakes hands with SKI and then with BIG AL.*

JEREMY
You take care, Big Al. Make sure Pappy here takes you to Rosie's place. All of you take care.

BIG AL
I feel like I'm losing my legs a second time.
> *(BIG AL looks heartbroken, then bursts out with a grin.)*

Hey, wait! I just remembered! Earl Ray left something I was supposed to read to you before you left!

> *BIG AL pulls a crumpled sheet of paper out of his pocket and smoothes it out.*

BIG AL
Earl Ray says:
> *(reading)*

"You're okay for a noncombat --"
> *(looks up and grins)*

Oh, no. Wait. That's not what this says. I'm sure that's what he <u>meant</u>, but what he <u>said</u> was, "for an honorary Marine."

JEREMY
> *(making air quotes)*

Thanks, "Earl."

BIG AL
"So promise me one thing, Shoff."

JEREMY
Anything you want, Earl.

BIG AL
"Get that tattoo."

> *They all burst out laughing, hooting, and hollering.*

JEREMY
You got it, Earl.

SKI
dYou are a lot like us, dyou know. Eet won't be the same around here without you, my dfriend.

JEREMY
And I'll never be the same without you guys.

> *JEREMY and PAPPY walk together toward stage right. When JEREMY reaches the curtain, he puts down his sea bag, turns around, snaps to attention, and salutes the MARINES on Q ward. They return the salute. JEREMY makes a sharp about face, picks up his sea bag, and exits through the curtain, glancing back at his friends one last time.*
>
> *Lights fade and go out, one at a time, stage right to stage left.*

<u>END OF ACT II</u>

The End

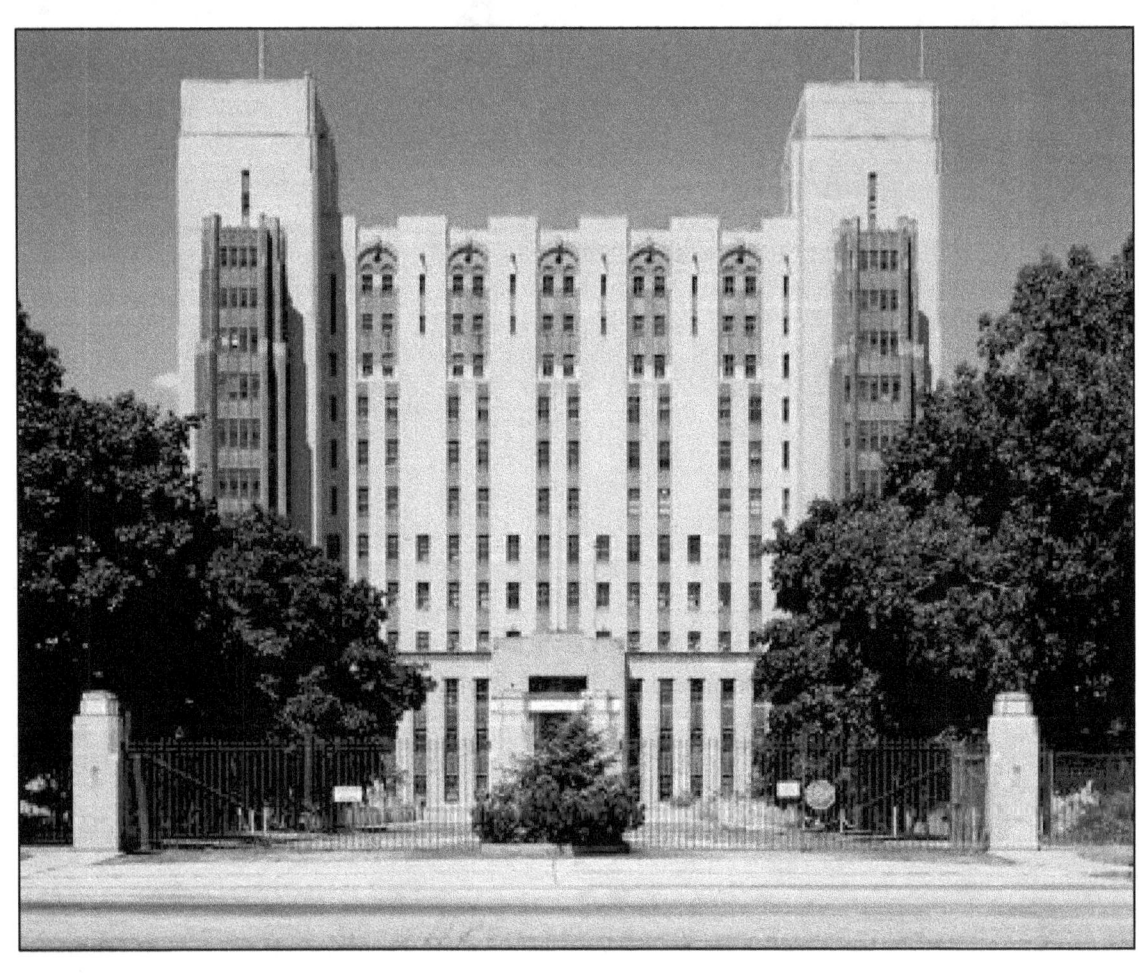

U.S. Naval Hospital, Philadelphia, PA, 1969

PURPLE HEARTS

based on the novel
How Can You Mend This Purple Heart
by
Terry L. Gould

adapted for readers theater by
Terry L. Gould and M.C. Nelson

To contact Terry Gould,
email:
purplescribe68@gmail.com

Cast Of Characters

Doc Miller:	Navy hospital corpsman. Age 20.
Ski:	Russian-born patient. USMC. Age 19.
Jeremy:	Patient. Navy. Age 19.
Earl Ray:	Patient. USMC. Age 19.
Dr. Donnolly:	Navy orthopedic surgeon. Mid 40s.
Miss Berry:	Navy Lt. Commander. Late 30s.
Bobby Mac:	Patient. USMC. Pt Cherokee. Age 22.
Moose:	Patient. USMC. Age 19.
Ski's Poppa:	Immigrant. Russian. Mid 50s.
Roger:	Patient. USMC. Age 19.
Admiral:	Officer with an attitude.
Big Al:	Patient. USMC. Age 20.
Pappy:	Patient. US Coast Guard. Age 27.
Bar Patron:	Any age bar patron.
Eva:	Bar owner. Early 30s.
Rosie:	Brothel owner. Early 30s.
Tiny:	Navy Chief Petty Officer. Mid-30s.
Hippie:	Female war protester. Early 20s.
Sgt. Pepper:	USMC war protester. Early 20s.
Dave:	Mafioso. Mid-40s.
Escort:	Call girl. Early 20s.
Off-screen Voices:	Can be read by any offstage actor.

Scene

U.S. Naval Hospital and other sites in Philadelphia, Pennsylvania, and Atlantic City, New Jersey.

Time

1969, early in the Vietnam War.

ACT I

SCENE 1

SETTING: *FOR NINE-ACTOR READERS THEATER CASTING AND SEATING CHART, SEE PAGE 3. For both acts, all scenes: nine seats are in a row from left to right. If six wheelchairs are available, they should be used for seats 1,2,3 and 7,8,9. The center three seats (4,5,6) should be chairs or stools. The NARRATOR sits off the stage, at either side. In front of each seat is a stand holding a copy of the script. If costumes are available, during the first act all patients (seats 1-3 and 7-9) wear pajamas; medics (seats 4-6) wear US Navy uniforms.*

AT RISE: *From stage left to stage right, seated are: empty, empty, EARL RAY, DR. DONNOLLY, MISS BERRY, DOC MILLER, SKI, JEREMY, empty.*

NARRATOR
The play *Purple Hearts* begins on Ward 2B, the Orthopedic Ward of the Philadelphia Naval Hospital, 1969. In an arc across the stage from the audience's left to right are: an empty wheelchair, JEREMY dozing in a wheelchair, a space for SKI's wheelchair, a stool for DOC MILLER, a small table, a stool where MISS BERRY is sitting, a small table with a battery operated drill on it, DR. DONNOLLY sitting on a stool, EARL RAY in a wheelchair, and two more empty wheelchairs. At rise, the lights come up on each seat, in order from stage right to stage left. DOC MILLER comes in pushing SKI in his wheelchair to the empty spot between JEREMY and the empty stool. Doc then sits on the empty stool.

DOC MILLER
Okay, Ski, Dr. Donnolly'll be in to see you in a little while. He's the one who put your legs back together. In the meantime, we'll get you another needle to help you relax.

SKI gives a thumbs up.

JEREMY (*waking*)
What's happening? Who are these people? Dear God, what is this place? Am I in Hell?

DOC MILLER
Easy, Shoff. You're not in Hell. Well, not exactly. You're in the Philly Naval Hospital. You're here 'cause you were in a car wreck three days ago and almost died. You needed the best orthopedist we've got, so they brought you here. You're in good hands with Dr. Donnolly. He treats the Marines back from Nam.

JEREMY
These guys here. That's who they are, aren't they? They're Marines who were wounded in Vietnam, aren't they? <u>Aren't they!</u> I should have been in Vietnam with them instead of joining the Navy. I should never have backed out of joining the Marines. I should have been one of them. I am so ashamed that I wasn't.
(MORE)

                        JEREMY (CONT'D)
That I took the easy way out. I don't deserve to be in the same
room with them. To be in their presence. Oh, God, I am so ashamed.

                *EARL RAY looks over and
                gives JEREMY the finger.*

                        EARL RAY
Noncombat motherfucker.

                        SKI
Felix Dawntay dJamnitzky.

                        JEREMY
What?

                        SKI
Felix Dawntay dJamnitzky. Allld my friends call me Skee.

                        JEREMY
Jeremy Shoff. All my friends just call me Shoff.

                        SKI
dYou look like sheet.

                        JEREMY
What?

                        SKI
dYou look like sheet.

                        JEREMY
You don't look much better. What happened to land you in here?
            (*pause*)
Maybe I shouldn't have --

                        SKI
Eet's okay. Eet's just that my leg, eet burns sometimes. Eet
was a land mine. My buddy tripped dthe wire. He took most of
dthe blast. Died instdantly.

                        JEREMY
Where're you from?

                        SKI
dNew Jersey.

                        JEREMY
No, really. Where're you from?

                        SKI
I was born in dRussia. Someday, I want to be ceetizen here.

                    DOC MILLER
Okay, Ski, here's that morphine for you. Let's see that bulldog
tattoo. You choose. Where should that bulldog get it this time?
How about right between the eyes?

                         SKI
I don't care. Just geeve eet to me.

                    DOC MILLER
How about you, Shoff? You need anything? If you do, just ask
for me. The name's Randy Miller, but you know us corpsmen; we
like to think we're more than glorified medics. Everyone here
just calls me Doc.

                       JEREMY
Yeah, Doc. As soon as you can.

                    DOC MILLER
You've got it. I'll be back in a little while to bring it and
check on you two. Oh! I almost forgot. You had a buddy who
came to see you before he shipped out. I think his name was Bill?

                       JEREMY
My best friend. He had more sense than to go out partying with
us the night we graduated, so he was spared being in the wreck.

                    DOC MILLER
He said to tell you the two in the back seat were sent to Aberdeen.
Two others are here, on a different ward, and are doing well.
But the driver, well, he didn't make it. And your friend must
know you well, because he said for you to not give us any trouble.

                  JEREMY (*laughing*)
Yeah. Like I would do that.

                    DOC MILLER
You need anything while I'm getting out the shots, Earl Ray?

                       EARL RAY
                (*gives DOC the finger*)
What the hell do you think, Doc?

                       JEREMY
You really from Russia, Ski?

                         SKI
dYep.

                       JEREMY
What's Russia like?

                         SKI
I don't dknow. We moved here when I was leetle. My parents let
me enlist. I am not a ceetizen yet. But someday, I hope.

                    DR. DONNOLLY
Hello, Ski. I'm Dr. Donnolly, and this is Lt. Commander Dorothy
Berry. Miss Berry is the head nurse for this floor and she's
going to help me take a look at you. I know this is going to
hurt, but you could have been paralyzed, Ski, and I need to see
what we have back there.
                         (*pause*)
It looks pretty good, considering. Unfortunately, we can't remove
that piece of shrapnel from the back of your throat. It's too
dangerous.

                         SKI
Eet doesn't hurt that much, sir.

                    DR. DONNOLLY
That's good to know. Now I need to take a look inside your legs.
If it gets to be too much, we'll stop. Just let me know.

                         SKI
Eeets okay.

                    DR. DONNOLLY
The shrapnel shattered both of your shin bones, so we attached
steel rods to them, leaving gaps in the bones between your ankles
and knees. As your shin bones grow, we can compress the rods
from out here. That assists the fusion. Right now we need to
change the dressings on your legs. It's going to be uncomfortable.

                    MISS BERRY
Are you doing okay, Ski?

                         SKI
Yes, ma'am. Eets okay.

                    MISS BERRY
Let me know if this gets to be too much, Ski. We've got all day.

                    SKI (*writhing*)
Eet's okay, ma'am.

                         JEREMY
Take my hand, Ski!

              SKI grabs JEREMY's hand.

                    MISS BERRY
Hold on, Ski. We're almost finished. Just two more. Can we get
him something, Doctor?

                    DR. DONNOLLY
Bring me a half dose of morphine, Randy. We're going to need to
change that dressing three times a day, Ski, so if it gets to be
too much at any time, just let us know.

SKI

Eets okay, sir.

JEREMY

I can't believe how you handled that, Ski. I couldn't have done it. Not one word from all that pain.

SKI

Eeet wasn't that bad. Not as bad as that fawcking land mine. Thanks for your hand. I hope I didn't squeeze too hard. I sure could use a cigdarette.

DOC MILLER

Sorry, Ski. You're not allowed to smoke right after a needle. You might drop your cigarette and burn yourself.

SKI

dWhat in the hell dwe supposed to do?

DOC MILLER (*laughing*)

Just ask for another needle. No tobacco after a shot, but unlimited morphine. We give it out like candy. Just ask.

DR. DONNOLLY

Randy, can you get me a sterile gown pack?

DOC MILLER

Yes, sir. Is it time, sir?

DR. DONNOLLY

Yes. Thanks, Randy. I think it's time. Is everyone ready?

MISS BERRY/DOC

We're ready.

SKI

Uh-oh, Shoff. It looks like dyou are dnext.

DR. DONNOLLY

Jeremy, now that your concussion is clear, we need to get this leg into traction. To do that, we have to pull your leg tight to keep the broken ends of your femur from scraping together or cutting into your thigh muscle. We'll insert this pin crossways through your shin bone, just below your knee. It's going to be uncomfortable, but it should only take a few minutes.

JEREMY

Oh, shit. Sorry, sir.

DR. DONNOLLY

It's okay. We're giving you a special pain medication that should help, which should last just a little longer than it will take us to finish.

I-1-6

NARRATOR
DR. DONNOLLY carries the drill over to stand in front of JEREMY, his back to the audience, holding the drill hidden between them. He then turns it on for a few moments.

JEREMY (*writhing*)
AAUGH!

Sobbing, Jeremy covers his face with his hands.

DR. DONNOLLY
Breathe, Shoff! Breathe now!
    (*pause*)
Sorry, Jeremy, just a couple of mechanical adjustments, and we'll be done. I know it hurt. I wouldn't want to have to go through it myself.

MISS BERRY
We'll have something ready for your pain in just a few minutes. In the meantime, I think we need to remove some of the glass from that cut in your head. Let's get that bandage off you.

NARRATOR
DOC MILLER Removes JEREMY's bandage.

JEREMY
How's it look, Doc?

DOC MILLER
Wow. Too bad these aren't diamonds. We could make a fortune.

JEREMY
I'm sorry I yelled like that, Ski. You set the bar too high.

SKI
I just dthink I'm used to it by now. Dyou should have heard me when the land mine exploded.

EARL RAY
He didn't hear anything, 'cause he's a noncombat motherfucker.

JEREMY
Okay. I've seen your hateful looks, and I've heard them call you Earl Ray, so let's get this over with, Earl. I'm Jeremy Shoff, radioman, US Navy. I'm here 'cause the night before I was supposed to ship out I got drunk and was in a car wreck.

SKI
Felix Dawntay dJamnitzky. Lance dCorporal, U.-S.-M.-C., first battalion, seventh dMarines. A bad land mine.

                            EARL RAY
Why don't you just give him your fucking serial number while you're
at it? Shit, you don't know what a fucking bad land mine is.
                    (*points at right leg stump*)
Bad land mine, my ass.

                            SKI
Just geeve eet a break, Earl.

                            EARL RAY
Hey, noncombat motherfucker, do you know what it's like to kill
somebody? I didn't think so. I can't believe I'm in here with a
noncombat sissy motherfucker. Of all the bullshit fucking things
to happen to me. You even smell like a noncombat motherfucker,
Shoff. Somebody get me some noncombat motherfuckin' air freshener.

                            SKI
Geeve eet a fauwcking break, Earl.

                            JEREMY
It's okay, Ski. Let it go. Maybe it makes him feel better.

                            EARL RAY
The only thing that would make me feel better is your noncombat
ass out of my sight.

                            JEREMY
Then have them move your ass over to another ward.

                            EARL RAY
Why you smart-ass motherfucker!

                            JEREMY
No more than you, Earl.

                            SKI
Okay, dyou two. Geeve eet a break. Why don't dyou two just keese
and make up?

                            EARL RAY
Noncombat motherfucker can kiss my ass.

                    Lights fade and go out,
                    one at a time, stage right
                    to stage left.

ACT I

SCENE 2

SETTING: *FOR NINE-ACTOR READERS THEATER CASTING AND SEATING CHART, SEE PAGE 3. For both acts, all scenes: nine seats are in a row from left to right. If six wheelchairs are available, they should be used for seats 1,2,3 and 7,8,9. The center three seats (4,5,6) should be chairs or stools. The NARRATOR sits off the stage, at either side. In front of each seat is a stand holding a copy of the script. If costumes are available, during the first act all patients (seats 1-3 and 7-9) wear pajamas; medics (seats 4-6) wear US Navy uniforms.*

AT RISE: *From stage left to stage right, seated are: empty, empty, EARL RAY, DR. DONNOLLY, MISS BERRY, DOC MILLER, SKI, JEREMY, BOBBY MAC.*

NARRATOR
As scene two begins on Ward 2B, from the audience's left to right there is an empty space for a wheelchair, JEREMY and SKI in their wheelchairs, an empty stool, a small table with a rotary dial phone and a folder on it, MISS BERRY sitting on a stool, a small table, DR. DONNOLLY sitting on a stool, EARL RAY in a wheelchair, and two more empty wheelchairs. At rise, the lights come up on each seat, in order from stage right to stage left. DOC MILLER comes in pushing BOBBY MAC in his wheelchair to the empty spot next to JEREMY and then sits on the empty stool.

DOC MILLER
Let's see here.
Not too bad for what could have happened. Says here you jumped on a live grenade to save your buddies. You could have lost your head.

BOBBY MAC
What makes you think I didn't?

DOC MILLER
'Cause I can still see it. Randy Miller. Everyone calls me 'Doc.'

BOBBY MAC
Bobby Mac Joyce. Nice to know you, Doc. I'd shake your hand, but you'd have to go to Nam to get it.

DOC MILLER
Well, you're in luck, Bobby Mac Joyce. You still have your thumb. The whole thing.

BOBBY MAC
Well, ain't that some shit. They told me on the chopper I lost my whole arm.
    (*to JEREMY*)
Hey, man. I can tell you ain't combat. What the fuck happened to you?

JEREMY
The name's Shoff. Car hit a bridge.

BOBBY MAC
That fucking car wreck kicked your ass.

JEREMY
Yeah. But it ain't shit compared to you guys.

BOBBY MAC
Yeah, well, ain't a fucking thing we can do about it now. They let you smoke in here?

DOC MILLER
Need to put 'em down, Bobby. I gotta get your vitals. Can't have the smoke messing up the numbers.

BOBBY MAC
Shit, Doc. Just fill in some numbers. I'm breathing, ain't I?

DOC MILLER
No can do, Bobby Mac. Give me your right arm so I can get your B.-P. Need anything for pain?

BOBBY MAC
Better get a couple more of those shots ready, Doc, I'll need more soon. I used to have two or three before breakfast in Nam.

DOC MILLER
Brag all you want, but I can tell you're not a junkie. You're in great shape and that's probably what kept you from being any worse.

BOBBY MAC
Any worse? Shit, this is heaven! Got me a hotel room, a bed with clean sheets, and somebody bringing me drugs all day and night. Don't get any better than this, man.

DR. DONNOLLY
Let's take a look in that eye socket, Bobby. It's looking pretty good. How's it feel?

BOBBY MAC
Like there's a hole where there shouldn't be a hole. It's kind of drafty.

DR. DONNOLLY
It won't be too long before we can fit you with a replacement.

BOBBY MAC (*laughing*)
In the meantime, I'll keep an eye out for you.

DR. DONNOLLY
That was absolutely terrible, Bobby. How're *you* doing, Ski?

SKI

Eet's okay, sir.

DR. DONNOLLY

We need to get another set of x-rays and see how well we're doing. I won't make another adjustment for a couple more days. Give you a little break.

SKI

Thdank you, sir. Eet doesn't hurt all that bad.

DR. DONNOLLY

Thank you, young man.
                    (to EARL RAY)
Your arm is starting to look a lot better, Earl. Soon, we'll be able to start measuring for your new arm.

EARL RAY

Yeah. I can hardly wait.

DR. DONNOLLY

Let me have a look at the rest of you.

EARL RAY

You mean what's left of me.

DR. DONNOLLY

We're going to have you walking before you know it, Earl.

EARL RAY

Easy for you to say. I've been here too long already.

DR. DONNOLLY

The past six months must seem like forever, Earl, but you're doing really well. You only need a couple more minor surgeries and we'll be able to get you out onto the rehab wards.

EARL RAY

Oh, yeah? I'm doing well compared to _what_?

DR. DONNOLLY

Look, Earl, I can't imagine how you feel. But I --

EARL RAY

No, you can't! Ain't nobody can know how I feel! Jesus H. Christ!

DR. DONNOLLY

Earl, that's not going to help you. I need you to be positive about this. _You_ need it, too.

EARL RAY

Gimme that needle, Doc. I need to escape this shit.

DOC MILLER
Here you go, Earl.

EARL RAY
That all you got?

DOC MILLER
That's it, Earl. I can't wait for this to put you out.

EARL RAY
Me, neither. Hey, noncombat motherfucker, what do you do in the Navy, scrub floors? Kiss my ass, noncombat motherfucker.

JEREMY
You kiss my ass, Earl. What do you want me to do, have 'em cut my legs off? You've got a lot of reasons to hate me, Earl. It's okay. I don't blame you. I'd hate me, too, if I were you. Or maybe I wouldn't. A lot of these guys in here are looking at life in a wheelchair, and they don't hate me. It's just you, Earl. You're the one full of hate, and you're always directing it at me.

EARL RAY
Fuck you, Shoff. Can't wait to get my ass out of here. Me and my girlfriend Jen, we'll pick up where we left off.

SKI
Dyou are verdy lucky guy. My girlfriend told me to djust be careful, and I never heard from her again.

EARL RAY
What was her name?

SKI
I don't dremember. My first time to get laid was in Nam.

EARL RAY
I never touched the stuff. Jen's the only one for me.

SKI
That's why dyou are very lucky.

EARL RAY
Yeah. We'll see how lucky I am. Hey, Shoff, you got a girl?

JEREMY
Not any more. And thanks for not calling me a noncombat motherfucker.

EARL RAY
Don't be so happy, Shoff. You'll always be a noncombat motherfucker to me. What'd she do, Shoff? Your girl?

I-2-12

JEREMY
She sent me a "Dear John" while I was in boot camp. Said we didn't have a lot in common anymore. I found out later she was screwing a guy at college who was getting an education and had a Corvette. I just keep trying to figure out why I wasn't good enough.

SKI
Sounds dlike you were pretty serious. How long deed you go with her?

JEREMY
Just over a year. I thought we were headed for the altar. She's the one who talked me out of joining the Marines with my best friend.

EARL RAY
That's life, man. Look at you now. A noncombat motherfucker laid up in here with me just twelve feet away. You join the Navy to see the world and what you get is a world of shit. And that girlfriend fucked you twice.

JEREMY
Say what?

EARL RAY
Your girl. She fucked you twice. She left you for some school boy on campus <u>and</u> she talked you out of being with your buddy in the Corps.

JEREMY
Yeah, Earl. That was my mistake.

NARRATOR
MISS BERRY answers the phone.

MISS BERRY
   (*into phone*)
2B.
   (*pause*)
Yes. He's here.
   (*pause*)
I understand. All I can do is ask.
   (*pause*)
Yes, hold on.

NARRATOR
MISS BERRY carries the phone to EARL RAY and holds the handset out to him as she continues to hold the base.

MISS BERRY
It's for you, Earl. It's Jennifer again. She's at the gate. Again. Please talk to her, Earl. Just talk to her. Just give her a chance.
      (MORE)

                          MISS BERRY (CONT'D)
She's been writing and calling you and coming here for almost a
year. She's proved to you that she hasn't given up on you and
isn't likely to. Please, give her a chance. Please.

                          NARRATOR
EARL RAY accepts the handset. MISS BERRY holds the base as he
looks at her, looks at the handset, and finally answers.

                          EARL RAY
Hello, Jen. It's me. Earl.
          (*pause*)
I love you, too, Jen, but you love another Earl. The old Earl.
I'm not the same person you knew before.
          (*pause*)
You don't understand. I know you've been talking with my mother
and you think you know how bad it is, but whatever it is you're
imagining, it's worse.
          (*pause*)
You think the two of you have it worked out? You really think
you're ready? Because I'm <u>not</u> ready, Jen. I'm just not.
          (*pause*)
You're the <u>only</u> thing keeping me sane, Jen, but I'm still not
ready. Did you ever think of that?
          (*pause*)
Okay, Jen. I give up. You can come in. Just ask for Miss Berry
when you get to the desk and give me a few minutes. I'll come.

                          NARRATOR
Earl hands the handset back to Miss Berry, who puts phone back on
table.

                          MISS BERRY
It'll be okay, Earl. I'll go take care of everything.

                          NARRATOR
Miss Berry exits behind screen.

                          SKI
Anything you want to talk about, before Jendifer gets up here?

                          EARL RAY
I don't think I'm ready, Ski. What is she going to think when
she sees a guy with one arm and no legs?

                          SKI
Eet'll be okay, Earl. She loves dyou and dyou are very lucky.

                          EARL RAY
Jesus. Why did I agree to this? I'm not who she thinks I am.

                          SKI
A dMarine is aldways ready, my friend. Eet will be fine. Dwe
are all with you.

I-2-14

EARL RAY
Thanks, Ski.

NARRATOR
MISS BERRY returns to the stage and sits on her stool.

MISS BERRY
Okay, Earl. Jennifer is the Solarium, whenever you're ready to join her there. Is there anything else I can do to help?

EARL RAY
No, ma'am. I can do this. All I have to do is get myself in there, let go of the chair, put my arm around her, and tell her that I love her. I can do this. Let go of the chair. Put my arm around her. Tell her --

DOC MILLER
You want me to give you a push, Earl?

EARL RAY
No. I have to do this myself. I have to.

NARRATOR
EARL RAY propels his wheelchair towards the screen using his one hand, talking to himself as he goes.

EARL RAY
Get myself in there. Let go of the chair. Put my arm around her. Tell her that I love her.

NARRATOR
As EARL RAY goes behind the screen, there is a loud crash and a thud.

EARL RAY (*shouting*)
Jen! Jen! Miss Berry! Doc! Come quick! Please! Help! Help!

NARRATOR
MISS BERRY and DOC rush behind the screen. DOC runs back out and grabs an empty wheelchair, pushing it behind the screen. MISS BERRY slowly pushes EARL RAY back to his place.

EARL RAY
Oh, Miss Berry. Jen. Jen. Is she going to be okay?

MISS BERRY
I think she'll be fine, Earl, but she's going to need a few stitches where she hit her head on the table as she fainted. Randy will take her down to the emergency room, and will let us know what the doctor says.

EARL RAY
I should never have let her see me. It's all my fault.

MISS BERRY
She was just surprised, Earl. That's all. She was just surprised. She'll be okay. Just give her some time.

EARL RAY
I should never have let her see what is left of me. I shouldn't have told her she could come up. I knew neither of us was ready.

SKI
Eeet will be okay when she comes back up, Earl. You two weel be fine.

EARL RAY
I don't think I can make it without her, Ski.

NARRATOR
DOC MILLER comes back on the ward, pushing the empty wheelchair back to its place.

DOC MILLER
She's doing fine, Earl. The doctor on duty wants her under observation for a couple of hours, and then he's going to send her back to the motel to rest. There was no serious injury, they just want to make sure. Her mother is going to come pick her up. She will call you as soon as she feels better. She promised.

EARL RAY starts hitting his one good arm on the arm of his chair.

EARL RAY
No she won't! I know she won't! Fuck 'em. Fuck all of 'em. I don't give a shit about any of 'em. I didn't need her letters in Nam and I sure as hell don't need her help now. She and her mother can kiss my ass! All of you can kiss my ass!

SKI
Did Dmarines help dyou in Nam, Earl?

EARL RAY
That's a stupid fucking question. Of course they did. We helped each other right up until some asshole medics thought it was a good idea to save my worthless life. That didn't help at all. Now. You got any more stupid fucking questions like that one?

SKI
Well, dMarines are going to help dyou now.

Lights fade and go out, one at a time, stage right to stage left.

ACT I

SCENE 3

SETTING: *FOR NINE-ACTOR READERS THEATER CASTING AND SEATING CHART, SEE PAGE 3. For both acts, all scenes: nine seats are in a row from left to right. If six wheelchairs are available, they should be used for seats 1,2,3 and 7,8,9. The center three seats (4,5,6) should be chairs or stools. The NARRATOR sits off the stage, at either side. In front of each seat is a stand holding a copy of the script. If costumes are available, during the first act all patients (seats 1-3 and 7-9) wear pajamas; medics (seats 4-6) wear US Navy uniforms.*

AT RISE: *From stage left to stage right, seated are: MOOSE, empty, EARL RAY, empty, empty, DOC MILLER, SKI, JEREMY, and BOBBY MAC.*

NARRATOR
It is several weeks later on Ward 2B. From the audience's left to right, BOBBY MAC, JEREMY, and SKI are seated in their wheelchairs, DOC MILLER is on a stool, there's a small table, two empty stools with a small table between them, EARL RAY in a wheelchair, an empty wheelchair, and then MOOSE in a wheelchair. As the lights come up on each seat in order, SKI, BOBBY MAC, and JEREMY are laughing.

SKI
Dyou believe that, Shoff, and I will keese your ass!

BOBBY MAC
Now ain't that some shit! The one thing we all got in common with Shoff is we all have an ass!

EARL RAY
Speak for yourself! I ain't got nothing in common with the noncombat motherfucker. He's just a chicken-shit Navy coward, that's what he is.

JEREMY
We've been over this, Earl. Ain't no way I can change a god-damn thing! You want to hate me for having my arms and legs, go ahead.

EARL RAY
I hate you for a lot of fucking reasons, Shoff. Your girlfriend was right. You ain't got what it takes to be in the Corps. I wouldn't want you near me in a Marine's uniform. I know your kind. You'd probably turn your back and run as soon as it got a little tough. Fuck you, Shoff!

JEREMY
Fuck you, too, Earl! And don't come to me when you need someone to help you stand on your own two feet.

                            EARL RAY
Why, you son-of-a-bitch, I ought to come over there and choke the
living shit out of you!

                            JEREMY
Well come on over if you think you're man enough!

                            EARL RAY
You motherfucker! C'mon, Shoff!
                    (*rolls his wheelchair over
                    and slams it into Jeremy's*)
Show me what you got!

                            JEREMY
I'm not going to hit you, Earl.

                            EARL RAY
You can't take a man with no legs and only one arm?
                    (*shakes his fist*)
What kind of a pussy are you?

                            JEREMY
I'm not going to fight you!

                            EARL RAY
You're a chicken shit! You can't hit a guy with no legs and one
arm? C'mon noncombat motherfucker! Here's your chance!

                        JEREMY (*shouting*)
I ain't going to hit you, Earl!

                            NARRATOR
DOC MILLER jumps off his stool and jerks EARL RAY's wheelchair
away from JEREMY, pushing it back into its place.

                            DOC MILLER
You stay right there, Earl! Jesus Christ! What's the matter
with you two? Let's see what the hell we've got here. Shit!
                    (*stands looking at Jeremy*)
Your leg is going to need stitches, Shoff. How's it feel inside?

                            JEREMY
It's okay, Doc. Sorry. I fell out of bed trying to get the shit
pot off the floor. Earl Ray just came over here to help me.

                            DOC MILLER
What?

                            JEREMY
Well, you know, I dropped it on the floor and I was just trying
to get it when I fell over the edge of the bed. You were really
busy and I --

EARL RAY

Next time, let <u>me</u> get the shit pot off the floor for you.

> *DOC MILLER shakes his head as he walks back and sits on his stool.*

BOBBY MAC

Now ain't that some shit! I thought I left all the bullshit back in Nam.

SKI

Just let eet go, man.

BOBBY MAC

I've let a whole lot worse shit go than this little spat.

EARL RAY

Damn, Shoff, that felt good.

JEREMY

Glad I could help.

EARL RAY

It ain't over, you know.

BOBBY MAC (*laughing*)

Oh, bullshit, Earl, just let it go. Where're you from, Shoff?

JEREMY

Missouri. How 'bout you?

BOBBY MAC

Barlow by-God, North Carolina. My old man's full-blooded Cherokee. Sent me off to the Marines to keep my ass out of trouble. Didn't work. Got into more shit in Nam than anybody. Got to where I didn't even want to go home between tours, but they made me. Wait 'til he sees me now.

JEREMY

You're old man's Cherokee? My great grandmother was Cherokee on my dad's side.

BOBBY MAC

Ain't that some shit! By God, life just got better. I'm lying next to a relative! We'll have us a by-God family reunion right here!

EARL RAY

Yeah. Let's just fucking celebrate.

JEREMY

Your dad coming up anytime soon?

                                BOBBY MAC
Shit. I don't think he even knows I'm in the States. Life ain't
so bad. It's all in how you look at it. Just don't give a shit.

                                JEREMY
I hear you. So you jumped on a live grenade? That takes balls.

                                BOBBY MAC
No balls at all, man. Just did what I was supposed to do.

                                JEREMY
Yeah. Well, not everyone always does what he's supposed to do.

                                BOBBY MAC
It was fucking nothing.

                                JEREMY
Well, I don't think it's nothing.

                                BOBBY MAC
How're you doing down there, Earl Ray?

                                EARL RAY
What's it matter to you?

                                BOBBY MAC
Hey, man. Just trying to check on who I'm sleeping with.

                                EARL RAY (*shouting*)
None of your fucking business, man.

                                MOOSE
Oh, for God's sake. Don't you guys <u>ever</u> shut up down there?

                                EARL RAY
Who the fuck are you? And who made you H-M-F-I-C?

                                MOOSE
I'm Moose Johnson and <u>I</u> made me Head Motherfucker in Charge!

                                EARL RAY
What the fuck kind of name is Moose?

                                MOOSE
A nickname. Got it my first tour in country. We were in thick
brush following an ambush. I heard rustling in the tall grass so
I opened fire with my M60. Shredded a water buffalo into a thousand
pieces. I took shit for a month. Got a tattoo on my left arm
with my new name.

                    BOBBY MAC, JEREMY, SKI,
                    and MOOSE all laugh.

                    EARL RAY
You got a left arm?

                    MOOSE
Not all of it. Lost part of it with the bottom half of my left
leg.

                    EARL RAY
You mobile?

                    MOOSE
Nope. Won't be for a while.

            *EARL RAY leans across
            empty wheelchair and
            quietly talks to MOOSE.*

                    SKI
                (to Jeremy)
Hee'll come around. He's just being a badass. Eet's what he
knows.

                    EARL RAY
Hey, noncombat motherfucker. Moose agreed with me.

                    JEREMY
Yeah? What's that, Earl?

                    EARL RAY
<u>I'm</u> the Head Motherfucker in Charge.

                    JEREMY
I never doubted it, Earl. At least we've got one thing in common.

                    EARL RAY
What's that?

                    JEREMY
We're both motherfuckers.

                    BOBBY MAC
You think?

                    EARL RAY
That new eye of yours is looking good, Bobby Mac. Even I can see
better now that you've got it. In fact, I could even see you had
a catheter bag when they brought you in, this time. Glad to see
that frag didn't get your dick.

                    BOBBY MAC
Yeah, man ain't no way with this club on my hand I could hold
onto that pitcher to piss in, and I couldn't ever find anybody to
hold my dick for me, either! Hey, Shoff. You ever watch that
show, "Laugh-In"?

JEREMY

Yeah, all the time.

BOBBY MAC

Well, you know how those Rowan and Martin guys sign off? Dan Rowan says to Dick Martin, "Say goodnight, Dick," and Dick Martin says, "Goodnight, Dick."

JEREMY

Yeah. They do it every time.

BOBBY MAC
(*looking at his crotch*)

Goodnight, dick.

*BOBBY MAC, JEREMY, MOOSE
and SKI laugh*

NARRATOR

The lights begin to fade and go out, one at a time, from the audience's left to right At a fourth of the way...

JEREMY (*sweetly*)

Goodnight, dick!

NARRATOR

Halfway across...

SKI (*laughing*)

Gootnight, deek.

NARRATOR

Three fourths of the way...

MOOSE (*roaring*)

Goodnight, water buffalo!

NARRATOR

And as the last light goes out...

EARL RAY

Goodnight, assholes.

ACT I

SCENE 4

SETTING: *FOR NINE-ACTOR READERS THEATER CASTING AND SEATING CHART, SEE PAGE 3. For both acts, all scenes: nine seats are in a row from left to right. If six wheelchairs are available, they should be used for seats 1,2,3 and 7,8,9. The center three seats (4,5,6) should be chairs or stools. The NARRATOR sits off the stage, at either side. In front of each seat is a stand holding a copy of the script. If costumes are available, during the first act all patients (seats 1-3 and 7-9) wear pajamas; medics (seats 4-6) wear US Navy uniforms.*

AT RISE: *From stage left to stage right, seated are: MOOSE, SKI's POPPA (BIG AL wearing a coat and cap over his pajamas), EARL RAY, DR. DONNOLLY, MISS BERRY, DOC MILLER, SKI, JEREMY, and BOBBY MAC.*

NARRATOR
It is some months later on Ward 2B. In an arc across the stage, from the audience's left to right, BOBBY MAC, JEREMY, and SKI are seated in their wheelchairs, DOC MILLER is on a stool, there's a small table next to him, MISS BERRY is on a stool with a small table with a certificate and a small box with a bow on it next to her, DR. DONNOLLY is on a stool, and EARL RAY and MOOSE are in wheelchairs, with an empty wheelchair between them.

DOC MILLER
Got any special plans for today, Ski?

SKI
I don't, but dwhat do dyou want to know for?

DOC MILLER
Oh, nothing really. Just want to know if you have anything going on.

SKI
Dwhat are you going to do? You can leef my legs alone.

DOC MILLER
I'm not going to do anything with your legs. Well, not right now.

SKI
Thden what do you want weeth me?

MOOSE
He wants you to sing for him.

JEREMY
Don't look at me, Ski. I don't know what he's talking about.

DOC MILLER
Ski no! Please don't sing.
(MORE)

DOC MILLER (CONT'D)
I've heard you and Shoff before, and believe me, I don't need that. But what I would like is for you to look fine!

SKI
Why? Are we going somewhere or do you want to keese me?

DOC MILLER
You're not my type, Ski. I prefer American women.

SKI
You wouldn't go back to Ameridican women once you had a Roosian woman.

DOC MILLER
Never! Roosian women can't come close to American women.

SKI
Just wait. I will set you up with a Roosian woman. A real woman. She'll take care of your young Ameridican ass.

DOC MILLER
She'll have to wait. Right now, I want you to get washed up and comb your hair.

SKI
What the hell eeze going on?

JEREMY
I don't know. Better do what Doc says though; he seems pretty serious about it.

EARL RAY
Yeah. Maybe he has an Ameridican woman set up for you.

SKI
(*grabbing at his crotch*)
Bdring her on, baby! I'll show her really good Roosian time.

BOBBY MAC
Maybe he can bring me one, too while he's at it. Ameridican or Roosian, I don't give a shit!

NARRATOR
DOC MILLER combs SKI's hair.

MISS BARRY
Ski, you look absolutely four-oh.

SKI
Thdanks. Meese Berry, what eeze going on?

MISS BARRY
I really can't say, Ski. Officer's oath.

I-4-24

NARRATOR
MISS BARRY quietly exits behind the screen.

SKI
What the hell eez going on? I don't like theese at all.

DOC MILLER
Nothing at all, Ski.

SKI
Bullsheedt! Dyou had better tell dme dnow.

BOBBY MAC
Better tell him, Doc. He just might make you date that Roosian woman!

DOC MILLER
Okay. Okay. I think we're all ready.

NARRATOR
MISS BERRY enters the ward with SKI'S POPPA.

SKI
Poppa!

SKI'S POPPA
(*Embracing Ski*)
Felix, my dboy. Eet has been so dlong. I love dyou my boy! I love dyou! Dyou are home.

SKI
Poppa. Oh, Poppa.

SKI'S POPPA
Look at dyour legs. What eeze all of this? What eeze this thing? They send me letter telling me you weel be fine. You don't look fine to me. Oooh, Felix, this eeze all my fault. If I hadn't let you go. If only I had listened to my heart. I knew some think would be bad. Oh, my boy, I am so sorry. Look what I have done to my only son. Theese doesn't look right to me, my boy. How can dyou come home like this? Eet eez so goot to see you! You must come home now, Momma eez waiting to see you.

SKI
It is so goot to see you, Poppa.
(*the two hug for a moment*)
I must dwait till I can walk again. dThen I can come home.

SKI'S POPPA
I know dyou can't come home right now, my boy, but your Momma can't wait to see you.

SKI
I know Poppa. Soon enough I weel come home.

SKI'S POPPA
I thdink they have a surprise for you, Felix.

SKI
What do you mean? What else could there be?

SKI'S POPPA
I don't know. They just make sure I was here this day.

NARRATOR
MISS BERRY seats SKI'S POPPA in the empty chair.

MISS BERRY
You sit over here, Mr. Jamnitzky.

MISS BERRY/DOC MILLER/DR. DONNOLLY/EARL RAY/BOBBY MAC/JEREMY/MOOSE,
(*singing*)
From the halls of Montezuuuma to the shores of Tripoli. We will fight our countries baaatles in the air on land and sea.

DR. DONNOLLY
Outstanding! Outstanding!

SKI
What eeze going on here? Dr. Donnolly you don't look right. You being court martialed?

DR. DONNOLLY
Not hardly, Ski. I'm here to let your father know he has a new son.

SKI/SKI'S POPPA (*in unison*)
Dwhat!

DR. DONNOLLY
That's right. Ski, it is with the greatest pride and the deepest honor that I have been selected to present this to you.
(*taking the certificate
from the table and reading
aloud*)
"It is hereby authorized by the President of the United States, Commander in Chief of the Armed Forces, that Felix Dante Jamnitzky, Lance Corporal, United States Marine Corps, from this day and all days forward, is entitled to all inalienable rights guaranteed to every citizen under the Constitution of the United States of America." The President has granted you citizenship. You're a U.S. citizen, Ski!

*A photo of an American
flag replaces the image of
the ward projected on the
screen.*

SKI'S POPPA
(*crying openly and hugging
DR. DONNOLLY*)
My boy is ceetizen? He eez really a ceetizen of America? You are such a great doctor!

SKI
(*holding the certificate
and looking down at his
cast-covered legs*)
Poppa. I am a ceetizen. A U.S. ceetizen. Poppa, eet has all been worth eet.

DOC MILLER
And we're not quite done yet. Got one last surprise for you, Ski, my man!

SKI
Dwhat eeze it now? You going to take me home weeth you?

DOC MILLER
No, it's even better than that.

SKI
Nothing could be better dthan getting out of here.

DOC MILLER
That will come in due time. Right now it's due time for something else.

SKI
Dwhy don't you guys just leef me alone?

EVERYONE ON STAGE
Laughter.

SKI
Am I een some kind of trouble?

NARRATOR
Dr. Donnolly takes a small box from the table and hands it to SKI.

DR. DONNOLLY
Not at all, young man. We're here to present this to you. The Order of the Purple Heart medal. It's for the sacrifice you made for our nation. Please wear it proudly.

NARRATOR
SKI takes the Purple Heart medal out of the box.

*An image of a Purple Heart
medal replaces the image
of the flag on the screen.*

MISS BERRY
It's not every day that I get to be a part of this. Most of the time it's given before you guys arrive here. Ski, thank you, and please do wear it with pride. Every one of you, wear yours with all the pride in the world.

SKI'S POPPA
Felix, dmy boy, I must geet home and tell your Momma. She dwill be so proud. Dwe will come to see you soon. Goot bye, my boy.

SKI
Gootbye, Poppa. I can't wait to see you and Momma soon.

NARRATOR
MISS BERRY leads SKI's POPPA off the stage as EARL RAY pulls his own box from his pocket and looks at it. He rolls over to SKI and shows it to him.

EARL RAY
You, me and all the others in here with this, this is who we are. Take a good look at it, man. Sometimes it feels broken.

SKI
Dwhat do dyou mean?

EARL RAY
Sometimes it feels like it's broken. You know, like it's all for nothing.

SKI
Dyou are djust feeling Jendeefer, man.

EARL RAY
Shit, I've been feeling this way long before that.

SKI
Well, I think eet's all about Jendeefer. Dyou should be proud of dyour Purple Heart.

EARL RAY
Yeah, that's what they keep telling me.

SKI
Who's dthey?

EARL RAY
Those dumb, fucking shrinks they make me go to, who else?

SKI
They know what they are talking about. You should leesten to them.

                        EARL RAY
They don't know a god-damn thing. Trying to tell me my two legs
and arm are worth this little piece of purple and brass. It ain't
why I joined the Corps. I just wanted to be like my old man. Be
a Marine, go to war and come home and just live out my life.
Nobody said I'd come back like this. And they think this Purple
Heart is supposed to make me feel better? They're the ones that
are out of their fucking minds.

                        SKI
Dyou shouldn't feel that way.

                        EARL RAY
Nobody tells me how to feel, Ski. Not even you.

            *Lights fade and go out,
            one at a time, stage right
            to stage left.*

ACT I

SCENE 5

SETTING: *FOR NINE-ACTOR READERS THEATER CASTING AND SEATING CHART, SEE PAGE 3. For both acts, all scenes: nine seats are in a row from left to right. If six wheelchairs are available, they should be used for seats 1,2,3 and 7,8,9. The center three seats (4,5,6) should be chairs or stools. The NARRATOR sits off the stage, at either side. In front of each seat is a stand holding a copy of the script. If costumes are available, during the first act all patients (seats 1-3 and 7-9) wear pajamas; medics (seats 4-6) wear US Navy uniforms.*

AT RISE: *From stage left to stage right, seated are: MOOSE, ROGER (BIG AL wearing a white sweatshirt over his head and pajama shirt), EARL RAY, DR. DONNOLLY, MISS BERRY, DOC MILLER, SKI, JEREMY, and BOBBY MAC.*

                NARRATOR
In an arc across Ward 2B, from the audience's left to right, are BOBBY MAC, JEREMY, and SKI, seated in their wheelchairs; DOC MILLER, an empty stool, and DR. DONNOLLY on stools; EARL RAY, an empty space, and MOOSE in their wheelchairs. As the lights come up, MISS BERRY is wheeling new patient ROGER into the empty space.

                MISS BERRY
        (*to ROGER*)
How are you feeling, young man?

                ROGER
Not bad, ma'am.

                MISS BERRY
I'm Miss Berry. Let me or Doc Miller know if you need anything. Dr. Donnolly will be up later to check on you.

                ROGER
Thank you, ma'am.

                EARL RAY
Hey Doc. What's the new guy got?

                BOBBY MAC
He looks like a giant turtle on its back with his head stuck out.

                DOC MILLER
Two broken femurs, two broken arms, cracked skull and busted pelvis, motorcycle. He was home on leave from A-I-T before going to Nam.

                SKI
        (*laughing at EARL RAY*)
A non-combat moderfucker.

                    EARL RAY
              (*glaring at JEREMY*)
Yeah, but he's a Marine.

                    MOOSE
What difference does it make? Makes no difference, man. We're
all here for the same reason. We got messed up and we gotta get
on with shit, that's all.

                    JEREMY
What's his name?

                    DOC MILLER
Roger George. Just made Lance before he went home.

                    JEREMY
              (*aside to SKI*)
Well, he may be a Marine, but at least he's noncombat.

                    DR. DONNOLLY
Roger, we need to have a talk about your legs. Your last set of
x-rays shows your two femurs are not healing properly. This body
cast is not working. If we continue as is, your legs will curve
inward. I'm recommending that we put a steel rod in each femur,
just like we did for Jeremy's leg. If you want to walk upright
again, I'm afraid we don't have any other choice.

                    ROGER
I understand sir. When can you do it?

                    DR. DONNOLLY
We'll need to do two separate surgeries at least a week apart.
I'll get them scheduled right away.
              (*to SKI*))
Good morning, Ski.

                    SKI
Goot morning, sir.

                    DR. DONNOLLY
How do your legs feel inside, Ski?

                    SKI
Not bad, sir. They haven't hurt too badly in a while now.

                    DR. DONNOLLY
That's excellent. You're coming along quite well.

                    SKI
Dthank you. Dr. Donnolly, dyou know those rods you put in Jeremy's
dleg and can put in Roger's, too, to help them heal? Can you put
those things in my dlegs, too?

DR. DONNOLLY
I'm sorry, Ski. No one has invented a procedure for shin bones. You need a hollow bone like the femur for that surgery. But we do have some really good news. Your legs are doing well enough we're going to remove the upper half of the casts. We'll remove them to just below your knees and we'll take the stabilizer bar out from between your legs, too.

SKI
Did dyou guys hear that?

EARL RAY/MOOSE/JEREMY/BOBBY
MAC cheer.

DR. DONNOLLY
And it gets even better. We're going to attach rubber heels to the bottom of both casts, so we can get you ready to stand up.

EARL RAY/MOOSE/JEREMY/BOBBY
MAC cheer louder.

SKI
dThank you, sir. dThank you.

NARRATOR
DR. DONNOLLY exits behind the screen, with DOC MILLER wheeling SKI after him. When DOC MILLER brings SKI back out, SKI has exchanged his white pants for blue and white striped pajama pants with white coverings below the knees only. He is holding crutches.

DOC MILLER
We're not going to try walking today, Ski. Just get you to stand up for a few minutes. It's been almost four months since you've been upright. We'll take it slow. You ready for this?

SKI
A dMarine eez aldways ready.

DOC MILLER
Alright. Grab these crutches. Here we go.

NARRATOR
DOC MILLER tries to help SKI out of his wheelchair with the crutches for support. As SKI tries to stand, he collapses to the ground with his arms over his head.

SKI
Eet got me! Corpsman! My dlegs! My dlegs! Corpsman! Over here! I've been heet. Corpsman! Corpsman!

EARL RAY
It's a flashback, Doc! He's having a flashback!

NARRATOR

DOC Miller cradles SKI in his arms.

EARL RAY

It's over, Ski. It's over. They can't get you here. It's over, Ski. The bastards can't get you here.

DOC MILLER
(*helping SKI back into his wheelchair*)

Oh God, Ski. I'm sorry. I'm so sorry. I should have held on to you. I'm sorry, Ski. This shot will help. I'm so sorry.

DR. DONNOLLY
(*rushing onto the ward*)

I got here as fast as I could, Randy. I came as soon as I heard about Ski. You couldn't have known. You did all you could.

DOC MILLER

No, sir. I let him down. I should have known it might happen. I let him down.

DR. DONNOLLY

Don't be so hard on yourself, Randy. No one can predict combat flashbacks. They just happen. We all do the best we can.

DOC MILLER (*weeping*)

Yeah, I guess so.

DR. DONNOLLY

How are feeling, Ski?

SKI

Nawt too bad.

DR. DONNOLLY

Ski, we need to take some X-rays right away. I have to see if anything serious is going on in there. That means we need to lift your legs up a bit. You ready to let us take a look?

EARL RAY

A Marine is always ready.

NARRATOR

DOC MILLER pushes SKI behind the screen, with DR. DONNOLLY following them.

SKI (*groggily*)

Damn dright. A dMarine eez always ready.

NARRATOR

After a pause, DR. DONNOLLY slowly returns.

DR. DONNOLLY
It's SKI's right leg, men. It was damaged pretty badly from his fall. He was bleeding internally and it couldn't wait. We had to amputate. I wanted to tell you myself so you'd be ready when he gets here.

NARRATOR
DOC MILLER slowly pushes SKI back into his place on the ward. The white "cast" on SKI's right leg is now covered by black from the knee down.

DOC MILLER
I'm so sorry, Ski. I'll make it up to you. I will. Somehow. I will.

NARRATOR
EARL RAY rolls over to SKI's wheelchair and takes his hand.

EARL RAY (*sadly*)
Welcome to the club, my friend. Welcome to the club.

> *The lights fade and go out, one at a time, stage right to stage left.*

ACT I

SCENE 6

SETTING: *FOR NINE-ACTOR READERS THEATER CASTING AND SEATING CHART, SEE PAGE 3. For both acts, all scenes: nine seats are in a row from left to right. If six wheelchairs are available, they should be used for seats 1,2,3 and 7,8,9. The center three seats (4,5,6) should be chairs or stools. The NARRATOR sits off the stage, at either side. In front of each seat is a stand holding a copy of the script. If costumes are available, during the first act all patients (seats 1-3 and 7-9) wear pajamas; medics (seats 4-6) wear US Navy uniforms.*

AT RISE: *From stage left to stage right, seated are: MOOSE, an empty wheelchair, and EARL RAY in wheelchairs; ADMIRAL (DR. DONNOLLY who has replaced his Navy uniform with the ADMIRAL's jacket and cap), a small table, MISS BERRY, a small table with a rotary dial phone on it, and DOC MILLER on stools; and SKI, JEREMY, and BOBBY MAC in wheelchairs.*

        NARRATOR
In an arc across Ward 2B, from the audience's left to right, are BOBBY MAC, JEREMY, and SKI, seated in their wheelchairs; DOC MILLER, MISS BERRY, and an empty stool; and EARL RAY, an empty wheelchair, and MOOSE in their wheelchairs. As the lights come up, SKI, BOBBY MAC, JEREMY and MOOSE are laughing.

        DOC MILLER
    (*into phone*)
Hello. Doc Miller, Ward 2B. Yes, just a sec. Hey, Earl! It's for you.

Who's calling me?

        DOC MILLER
Don't know. She wouldn't say.

        BOBBY MAC
Hot damn! I'll bet it's that Roosian woman.

        SKI
Give him the phone, Doc!

        NARRATOR
DOC MILLER carries the phone down to EARL RAY.

        EARL RAY
No need to leave it, Doc. This won't take long.
    (*into phone*)
Hello?
    (*pause*)
Oh, hi, Jen, I thought it might be you.
    (*pause*)
No need to be sorry. You didn't do anything anyone else wouldn't have done.
        (MORE)

EARL RAY (CONT'D)
(*pause*)
I didn't mean that.
(*pause*)
Yeah, I've been doin' a lot of thinking, too. I'm not sure trying again just now is a good idea.
(*dropping the phone*)
Son of a bitch!

NARRATOR
DOC MILLER picks up the phone and hands it back to EARL RAY.

EARL RAY
(*into phone*)
Sorry, Babe.
(*pause*)
Yes, I guess I did call you, Babe.
(*pause*)
I don't think coming to see me again is a good idea, Jen.
(*pause*)
You know why, Jen. I need a lot of time. A lot more time.
(*pause*)
Yeah, I'm getting your letters, Jen. I just don't feel like writing.
(*pause*)
I can't call you, not for a while.
(*pause*)
Okay, Jen. Okay. Bye.

SKI
Dyou are a dlucky guy, Earl. She eez a special woman, dyou know. Dyou should call her back.

EARL RAY
Yeah, some day. Some day when I'm feeling lucky. Not today.

MISS BERRY
You really should call her back someday, Earl.

EARL RAY
Yeah. Maybe, someday.

MISS BERRY
Okay then, everyone, let's get this inspection over with. It's too bad Roger's down in Post-Op and has to miss the excitement, because in that full-body cast, at least I'd be able to count on <u>one</u> of you to behave himself. The rest of you, I'm not so sure about. I know it's asking a lot, but <u>please</u> be on your best behavior today. This shouldn't take long and everything will be back to normal. Wish me luck. I'll be back up here with the brass in a few minutes.

NARRATOR
MISS BERRY exits behind the screen.

                              EARL RAY
Hey, Doc.

                              DOC MILLER
Yeah, what is it, Earl?

                              EARL RAY
We know the brass is coming up, but who is it?

                              DOC MILLER
This is the **big** guy. The admiral from Norfolk headquarters.

                              SKI
I've never seen an admeeral. I don't think they are allowed in Nam!

                              EARL RAY
Non-combat motherfuckers, all of 'em.

                              JEREMY
Just like me.

                              EARL RAY
No, not quite like you. At least you went through boot camp. These guys wouldn't know a boot if it kicked 'em in the ass.

                              BOBBY MAC
Ain't that some shit. We must be real important if an admiral is coming.

                              EARL RAY
Yeah. We're supposed to think they give a shit.

                              NARRATOR
The ADMIRAL and MISS BERRY come in and walk down the line of wheelchairs. The ADMIRAL stops when he gets to EARL RAY, who is staring down at his left half-leg. None of the patients are saluting. Only EARL RAY is singled out.

                              ADMIRAL
Where's your salute, young man?

                              NARRATOR
EARL RAY doesn't move.

                              ADMIRAL
I said, where's your salute, young man?

                              NARRATOR
EARL RAY straightens up as much as he can, and salutes with his right hand. He never looks at the ADMIRAL.

JEREMY
(to the ADMIRAL)
Are you shittin' me?

SKI/EARL RAY/BOBBY MAC
Holy shit!

ADMIRAL
(to JEREMY)
What is it that you have to say to me, young man?

JEREMY
With all due respect sir, I think you're the one who should be saluting him.

ADMIRAL
What's your name, sailor?

JEREMY
Shoff, sir. Jeremy Shoff.

ADMIRAL (furiously)
You're up for Captain's Mast, Shoff, as soon you're able.

NARRATOR
The ADMIRAL storms off the ward with MISS BERRY following him. When the doors close behind them, Ward 2B erupts in cheers.

SKI
Holy shdit! What deed you do, man?

EARL RAY
That was fucking unbelievable, Shoff!

JEREMY
I can't believe he would come in here and expect you guys to salute him. Who the hell does he think he is?

BOBBY MAC
Shoff, you are beaucoup dinky dow! You're a crazy motherfucker! You got balls as big as that brass's ribbon rack!

JEREMY
I wouldn't know, man. Right now, I can't find 'em.

MOOSE
You are in deep shit, my friend.

EARL RAY
Shoff, you're all right by me. Non-combat motherfucker or not, I can't believe you did that.

                              SKI
                    (giving JEREMY a salute)
I dsalute dyou, Shoff!

                            JEREMY
Thanks, Ski, but I've got my ass in big trouble and it's Miss
Berry I'm worried about. I don't know what she's going to say to
me.

                           BOBBY MAC
Ain't that some shit! Beaucoup dinky Dow, Shoff! You're a crazy
mother fucker!
                    (farting loudly.)
Keep talking admiral, we'll find you.

                    Everyone laughs.

                            MOOSE
Shoff is right, you know. We don't have to salute those bastards!
What are they going to do? Send us to Nam?

                     EARL RAY/SKI/BOBBY MAC
Damn right! Hell yes!

                          MISS BERRY
I will deny that I ever said this, but, thank you, Jeremy.
                    (to everyone)
Well! Now that that's over with, anyone going to P-T, make sure
you wrap those limbs tight. We don't want any swollen limbs in
the morning.

                          DOC MILLER
Yeah, the guys down in physical therapy won't be too happy if
you're a mess when you come back tomorrow.

                           EARL RAY
What do they care? Those guys are like gorillas, anyway. Swollen
stumps don't slow them down.

                            MOOSE
                    (flexing the muscle in his
                     left arm)
It takes gorillas to make gorillas.

                             SKI
They push hard, but they can't push us hard enough. Eet feels
goot to be lifting weights again.

                          MISS BERRY
That's the attitude, you guys. The faster you get stronger, the
quicker you can transfer to the rehab wards and then on your way
home. Out there, you'll be on your own. All you will have is
each other.

DOC MILLER
If I ever get into a fight, I want you guys on my side.
(everyone chuckles)
We'll see you in the morning.

NARRATOR
MISS BARRY and DOC MILLER exit behind the screen.

EARL RAY
C'mon Shoff. Get that rickshaw of yours and let's go have a smoke.

JEREMY
It's raining out, man. Haven't you noticed?

EARL RAY
We ain't going out. We're going to the room.

*JEREMY begins to fidget
and wring his hands.*

BOBBY MAC
Relax, Shoff. We ain't taking you to the fucking gallows.

JEREMY
Don't be so sure. I've heard you and the others share stories about the solarium. It's sacred ground for you guys. I don't belong in there. Dr. Donnolly made it off limits to anyone not a patient on 2B. And you guys made it off limits to noncombat motherfuckers like me.

EARL RAY
If we invite you, you're going in.

JEREMY
I don't know, Earl. It's not right for me to join you guys in there. I don't deserve to be in that room with you guys. Shit, I don't deserve to be on the same ward with you.

BOBBY MAC
Bullshit, Shoff. Don't you dare fucking say no to us. Hey, Ski, Shoff's coming. You want to join us?

SKI
I dwouldn't meesse eet for nothing. Somebody go call down to the rehabs and get Big Al to come up. He dwon't want to meese this.

*Stage lights fade and go
out, one at a time, stage
right to stage left.*

ACT I

SCENE 7

SETTING: *FOR NINE-ACTOR READERS THEATER CASTING AND SEATING CHART, SEE PAGE 3. For both acts, all scenes: nine seats are in a row from left to right. If six wheelchairs are available, they should be used for seats 1,2,3 and 7,8,9. The center three seats (4,5,6) should be chairs or stools. The NARRATOR sits off the stage, at either side. In front of each seat is a stand holding a copy of the script. If costumes are available, during the first act all patients (seats 1-3 and 7-9) wear pajamas; medics (seats 4-6) wear US Navy uniforms.*

AT RISE: *From stage left to stage right, seated are: MOOSE, BIG AL, and EARL RAY in wheelchairs; three empty stools with plants on them; and SKI, JEREMY, and BOBBY MAC in wheelchairs.*

NARRATOR
In an arc across the solariium, from the audience's left to right, are BOBBY MAC, JEREMY, and SKI, seated in their wheelchairs; three empty stools with plants on them; and EARL RAY, an empty space, and MOOSE in their wheelchairs. As the lights come up, SKI, BOBBY MAC, JEREMY and MOOSE are laughing.

MOOSE
Did you guys call down to Q ward for Big Al?

BIG AL
Did I hear my name?

NARRATOR
BIG AL rolls in and takes his place in the half circle.

MOOSE
Man, that didn't take long. Glad you could join us.

BIG AL
I wouldn't miss this for the world.

EARL RAY
How's everything out on the rehabs, Big Al?

BIG AL
Same old shit, Earl. Be glad when you get out there. I need somebody to beat at Spades.

EARL RAY
You couldn't beat me in a chair race. I haven't heard when they're moving me back out, but when they do, I'll race you down the ramps.

BIG AL
You got a deal.

EARL RAY (*flexing his right arm*)
And I don't need a head start either.

                         BIG AL
I wouldn't have it any other way.

                         BIG AL
                    (to Jeremy)
Hey, Shoff. Earl Ray says you don't like being called a non-combat
motherfucker. Don't blame you. Earl Ray should worry more about
himself instead of looking around at what everybody else has or
doesn't have. Ain't that right, Earl Ray?

                         EARL RAY
I'm the one that said we ought to bring him in here, ain't I?
Don't mean shit to me anymore what anybody's done. Nothing means
shit to me anymore.

                         SKI
Dwhat about Jendeefer?

                         EARL RAY
What about Jendeefer? Jennifer ain't shit either. I'm just
going to get me a whore to live with when I get out of here.
Somebody that doesn't know shit about me and doesn't want to know.

                         MOOSE
Okay. Okay. Let's save it for later. Big Al, did you bring
that care package from your buddies in Nam?

                         BIG AL
Absolutely! And a surprise! I brought a bottle of Jack!

                         NARRATOR
BIG AL pulls a bottle of Jack Daniels from under his pajama top
and a small bundle from behind his back and opens it. From the
bundle, he pulls out a couple of Thai sticks, a short letter, and
a couple of Polaroid pictures. As the guys pass the pictures and
joints around, EARL RAY opens the Jack Daniels, takes a swig and
hands two of the photos to JEREMY.

                         EARL RAY
Ain't that a pretty sight? Take it in Shoff. Take as much time
as you need, man. You look at it long enough you may not give a
shit either?

                         NARRATOR
JEREMY looks, hands the pictures to SKI, then takes a swig of the
Jack and hangs his head.

                         EARL RAY
You wanted to be here, Shoff. If you don't like it, now's your
chance to leave.

                         JEREMY
I ain't leaving, Earl.
                         (MORE)

JEREMY (CONT'D)
A couple of pictures with dead people ain't going to make me go. I just don't want you to hate my guts. I can't change who I am and what's happened.

EARL RAY
I don't hate your guts, Shoff. I just hate who you are. I hate every motherfucker out there. So don't think you're so special. If I didn't want you in here, believe me, you wouldn't be in here.

JEREMY
You guys don't know what it means for me to be in this room.

SKI
Yes, dwe do. We just weesh you dwere a dMarine.

MOOSE
So. We've talked it over Shoff. We think you're all right for a non-combat motherfucker. We all agree. You're in here because we want you in here. Shoff, we're making you an honorary Marine!

JEREMY sits up straight and smiles.

EARL RAY
Just because you stood up to that admiral doesn't mean you're one of us, Shoff. It just means we don't mind having you around.

JEREMY
I gave up my chance to be one of you a long time ago. But if it's all right with you guys, when I get out to the rehabs, I'll get me a tattoo-Honorary U.-S.-M.-C.

EARL RAY
I'll go with you and make sure it ain't too big. And it can't be where anyone can see it.

JEREMY
I wouldn't care if it was on the top of my head.

SKI
Dyou see. dThat is why we like you.

BOBBY MAC
Now, ain't that some shit! We got us a genuine honorary by-God fuckin' Marine! And a relative to boot! Don't get no better than this man!

NARRATOR
JEREMY passes BOBBY MAC the bottle of Jack and BOBBY MAC takes a big swig.

EARL RAY
Don't get too cocky, Shoff. You'll always be a noncombat motherfucker. So don't forget it. Bobby Mac, hand me that Jack.

NARRATOR
The guys pass around the Jack Daniels and there is a quiet pause. EARL RAY takes a big drink from the bottle.

EARL RAY
It's happening you know.

MOOSE
What's that?

EARL RAY
People are beginning to hate us.

MOOSE
Ain't a damn thing we can do about it.

EARL RAY
Yeah, but how can they hate a guy with no legs? What the fuck do they know?

MOOSE
Fuck 'em. We don't owe them shit anyway.

BOBBY MAC
Ain't that some shit. Their day will come.

EARL RAY
You think they ever think they might owe us something? Fuck no they don't. They're spitting on our guys coming home for Christ's sake!

MOOSE
Take it easy, Earl. You don't want to get worked up over those assholes.

BOBBY MAC
Moose is right, Earl. They ain't shit and won't ever be shit to us.

EARL RAY
If I had my legs, I'd track every one of them down and kill those fucking long hairs with my bare hand.

MOOSE
If I had my leg and my arm, I'd just go home and start all over.

EARL RAY
You mean you'd join the Corps and go back to Nam? That's bullshit.

MOOSE

No. I didn't say that. I said I'd start all over again. Just like I'm going to when I get my arm and leg and get out of here.

EARL RAY

It ain't the same.

MOOSE

I know it ain't the same. But it's what we got and we got to get used to it.

EARL RAY
(*points at his left stump*)

This is what we got, huh? I'm supposed to feel lucky because I've got my cock and that cheap fucking Purple Heart? Bull shit.

MOOSE

It's what we got, Earl. That and each other. You think I can do this alone? We all need someone's help, someone we can count on.

EARL RAY

I don't need anybody's help.

MOOSE

That ain't that what the Corps drilled into our thick heads.

EARL RAY

That's different.

MOOSE

No difference at all, Earl. Remember your first real combat? Man, I do. All the rah-rah in the world and I was still scared shitless. Well, I'm scared shitless now, my friend.

BOBBY MAC

Got to look at what you have, Earl. Not at what you used to have.

EARL RAY

You're right, Moose. Ain't nothing different about any of it. But I did the right thing, you know.

MOOSE

You know you did, Earl. All of us did.

EARL RAY

Yeah, but Jesus, look at me. You know, I still can't believe it. If I could only go back, get another chance, like it never happened.

MOOSE

It's okay, Earl. We all feel that way sometimes.

I-7-45

EARL RAY
What the fuck am I going to do? A man with no legs? One arm? You call this a man?

MOOSE
You're a whole lot more of a man than anybody, Earl. You're more of a man than any fucking long hair out there. You got to be proud of what you did in Nam.

EARL RAY
Yeah, well, fuck the war. And fuck the medals. Big fucking deal. Pieces of cloth and cheap tin that don't mean shit. They can't give me back my arm, my legs god dammit.

SKI
Dyou should be proud of dyour medals. Dyou deed --

EARL RAY
I know what I did. I killed enough of those fuckers to protect this country for a century. And what do I get? Salute the brass. Sit tall in your wheelchair. Be proud of what you did for your country. The Marine Corps builds men. Semper Fi. Bullshit. Simple fucking bullshit.

SKI
No matter dwhat, Earl, you got us.

EARL RAY
It was the right thing to do, right? What else could I have done? It's what I wanted, to be a Marine. Now, I just count my blessings. At least I have my cock. Both eyes are perfect, right? No shrapnel to the head or face. Man, how fuckin' lucky can I be? I'm still alive, right? So what's my bitch? Fuck the legs. Fuck the arm. Semper Fi, my ass. The Marine Corps builds stumps.

MOOSE
It's okay, Earl. This is life now. Anything you want, you know we're here.

EARL RAY
You think it's that easy, huh?

MOOSE
No. It ain't easy, Earl. Not for any of us.

EARL RAY
It's real easy for the non-combat motherfucker. Ain't that right, Shoff?

MOOSE
We all got shit to deal with.

                        JEREMY
It's okay, Moose. There's nothing I can say. Not to Earl, not
to you, or Ski, not to anybody. But if I had it to do over again,
I probably wouldn't be here right now. Who knows what would have
happened? What's done is done, Earl. For what it's worth, backing
out of the Marines was the most chicken-shit thing I've ever done.
And I'll regret it for the rest of my life. But no matter what
you think about me, you can count on me anytime.

                        EARL RAY
Count on you? For what? To piss me off? To remind me of all
the noncombat motherfuckers out there? To remind me how lucky I
am? Ski keeps telling me how lucky I am. You're the lucky one,
Shoff. Lucky I didn't kill you. Lucky you got both arms. And
lucky you've got your legs. On the day you <u>walk</u> out of here,
Shoff, stop and think how lucky you are.

                        JEREMY
I wouldn't call it luck, Earl.

                        EARL RAY
Then what do you call it?   Fate?

                        JEREMY
No, I call it shame.

            Lights fade and go out,
            one a time, stage right to
            stage left.

ACT I

SCENE 8

SETTING: *FOR NINE-ACTOR READERS THEATER CASTING AND SEATING CHART, SEE PAGE 3. For both acts, all scenes: nine seats are in a row from left to right. If six wheelchairs are available, they should be used for seats 1,2,3 and 7,8,9. The center three seats (4,5,6) should be chairs or stools. The NARRATOR sits off the stage, at either side. In front of each seat is a stand holding a copy of the script. If costumes are available, during the first act all patients (seats 1-3 and 7-9) wear pajamas; medics (seats 4-6) wear US Navy uniforms.*

AT RISE: *From stage left to stage right, seated are: MOOSE, ROGER (with white hooded sweatshirt covering his head), and EARL RAY in wheelchairs; DR. DONNOLLY, MISS BERRY, and DOC MILLER on stools; and SKI, an empty wheelchair, and BOBBY MAC in wheelchairs.*

NARRATOR
It is the patients' last day on Ward 2B. In an arc across the solariium, from the audience's left to right, are BOBBY MAC, an empty wheelchair, and SKI, seated in their wheelchairs; an empty stool, MISS BERRY, and DR. DONNOLLY on stools; and EARL RAY, ROGER (wearing the white hooded sweatshirt over his pajama shirt and head), and MOOSE in wheelchairs. As the lights come up, DOC MILLER is walking over to SKI.

MOOSE
Hey, Doc. You're sure looking damn sharp. You getting ready for a big night out?

DOC MILLER
Nope. It's just another Friday night for me. Besides, with you guys graduating to the rehab ward, I'm taking two weeks' leave starting tomorrow. Remember? Got an early flight.

SKI
No one deserves eet more than you.

DOC MILLER
Well, I don't know about that, but I understand they're sending you guys all out to the rehabs before I get back. You've done great. And remember. Once you're out there, you have to take care of each other.

ROGER
Ain't none of us could have made it without you.

DOC MILLER
Thanks. I know I couldn't have made it through some of the days if it hadn't been for you guys, too. If I'm lucky, maybe I can look you guys up when I get back.

EARL RAY
What do you mean when you get back? How much time off did they give you?

DOC MILLER
You know, the usual two weeks.

I-8-48

BOBBY MAC
Give _me_ two weeks leave and you'll never see my ass in here again.

Everyone laughs.

EARL RAY
Make sure you come out to the rehabs and find us when you get back.

DOC MILLER
Oh, I think you will all be long gone and home by then, my friends.

SKI
Dwhat do you mean, Doc?

DOC MILLER
I got my orders. I volunteered and I'm going to Vietnam. I owe it to you, Ski. I'm going to Nam.

SKI
Sawnoffabeetch.

NARRATOR
Everyone sits quiet. EARL RAY looks around the ward. DOC MILLER shakes everyone's hand, says goodbye and exits.

DR. DONNOLLY
Your being here has been a special time for all of us, not just for Randy. It takes a special person to do what you guys have done, and it has been my honor to be your doctor and surgeon. As I told each one of you, you're healing has only begun. Don't miss a day of physical therapy and if you do nothing else, keep every single appointment with your psychiatrists. They're going to help you get through the next few months and ready to go home.

SKI
Thdank you, Dr. Donnolly. Dyou are the best.

DR. DONNOLLY
(*shaking SKI's hand*)
Thank you, Ski. And let me say again, welcome to America.

SKI
(*sitting up tall in his wheelchair*)
My Poppa is so proud of dyou. He still thinks dyou did it.

DR. DONNOLLY
It was one of my most treasured moments with you guys. I'll never forget it.

MOOSE
We'll give Ski another celebration once we're all out on the rehabs. Big Al and Jeremy are already out there, making plans.

BOBBY MAC

Great! We'll have that by-God family reunion, too!

EARL RAY

You won't think it's so great once we get out there.

BOBBY MAC

We'll just have to make it great then. C'mon, guys. Let's get out of here and make room for the incoming.

DR. DONNOLLY

You men can come back up here anytime. We would be honored to see you.

BOBBY MAC
(*spreading his eyelids,
displaying his glass eye*)
I'll keep an eye out on these guys for you.
(*laughter*)

MISS BERRY
(*putting her hand on EARL
RAY's shoulder*)
It's been a long journey to this point. You're going to need each other on the rehab ward. Take care of each other.
(*choking up*)
I'm going to miss all of you.

ROGER

Even me, Miss Berry?

MISS BERRY (*laughing*)

No, Roger. Not you. You're not going anywhere just yet. That's just wishful thinking on your part.

ROGER (*laughing*)

Just thought I'd ask. You never know what the gorillas might be able to do to rehab a man in a full-body cast. And you know more bodies will be coming in soon, to fill all the rest of these beds.

*The lights fade and go
out, one at a time, stage
right to stage left. As
last light goes out...*

EARL RAY

When is this shit ever going to stop?

<u>END OF ACT I</u>

ACT II

SCENE 1

SETTING: *FOR NINE-ACTOR READERS THEATER CASTING AND SEATING CHART, SEE PAGE 3. For both acts, all scenes: nine seats are in a row from left to right. If six wheelchairs are available, they should be used for seats 1,2,3 and 7,8,9. The center three seats (4,5,6) should be chairs or stools. The NARRATOR sits off the stage, at either side. In front of each seat is a stand holding a copy of the script.*

If costumes are available, during the second act MOOSE, BIG AL, EARL RAY, SKI, and BOBBY MAC wear USMC uniforms. JEREMY, TINY, and DR. DONNOLLY wear US Navy uniforms; PAPPY wears a US Coast Guard uniform. The actor in seat 5 wears 1960s hotpants; the actor in seat 6 wears dark pants and an open necked shirt. Accessories for actors in seats 4,5,6 vary from scene to scene, to delineate their roles.

AT RISE: *From stage left to stage right, seated are: MOOSE, BIG AL, EARL RAY, PAPPY, empty, empty, SKI, JEREMY, BOBBY MAC.*

NARRATOR
By the time the second act opens, the patients have progressed to rehab Ward Q. In an arc across the stage from the audience's left to right are: BOBBY MAC in a wheelchair, an empty wheelchair, SKI in a wheelchair, three empty stools with footlockers between them, and EARL RAY, BIG AL, and MOOSE in wheelchairs. The lights come up on each seat, in order, as JEREMY enters wearing his white Navy uniform. He is limping and carrying a half-full sea bag.

BOBBY MAC
Well, looky here! My blood relative all dressed up and playing Navy! I didn't recognize you Shoff. You getting ready for that by-God family reunion? Or is that admiral after your ass?

JEREMY
I only wear it when I have to, Bobby. And the admiral probably <u>is</u> after my ass.

SKI
dWhat do you mean, you wear it only when you have to?

JEREMY
They gave me a temporary light-duty assignment in Special Services. An unbelievable desk job.

MOOSE
They may as well make it permanent. You still got a lot of P.-T. left.

II-1-51

JEREMY
Yeah. I'm going to stay here with you guys for as long as I can.
My first medical review board gave me three more months here.

SKI
dWhat do you do in Special Services?

JEREMY
You won't believe it. I'm in charge of the party desk! Well,
that's what I call it. This is the biggest personnel mistake the
Navy ever made. But for you guys, it's a miracle.

BIG AL
You're in charge of a party desk? We've hit the jackpot!

JEREMY
You got that right. It's clam bakes, picnics, and Welcome Home
parties sponsored by local V.-F.-Ws, American Legion posts, and
even a brewery.

BOBBY MAC
Well, when do we start?

JEREMY
Not for a couple of weeks. We're just now getting things lined
up. Man is it good to see you guys. They sent me to M Ward while
I've been waiting for you to get out here to the rehabs. Mind if
I bunk here?

EARL RAY
You got two good arms and two good legs, Shoff, so get your ass
on the top bunk next to the shithouse. I got the bottom bunk
next to yours and Big Al has the bottom bunk next to me. If you
don't like where we put you, then move back to the other ward.

JEREMY
This is fine with me, Earl. And the shithouse doesn't bother me
either.

EARL RAY
We didn't put you there to piss you off. We want you close to
the shithouse in case one of us needs you to wipe his ass.

JEREMY
Don't count on it.

EARL RAY
I knew I couldn't count on you, Shoff. Not even to wipe my ass.

JEREMY
Okay, Earl. I'll wipe your ass if you need me to. But don't
expect me to pull you out of the shitter if you fall in.

EARL RAY
Fuck you, Shoff. Look around you, man. We're all in the shithouse already.

JEREMY
This ain't so bad. It's better than 2B.

EARL RAY
Says you. We've got no morphine out here.

JEREMY
Is the pain that bad, Earl?

EARL RAY
It's always that bad. Welcome to Q.

MOOSE
Welcome to Q, Shoff! You got that bunk because we don't want someone we don't know sleeping too close to us. Besides, you can stand watch over this end of the ward from up there.

JEREMY
No one gets past that you don't want to get past.

MOOSE
Ski has the bunk over there and Big Al and Bobby Mac have those two bunks. Glad to have you here, Shoff.

BOBBY MAC
Just one big happy family! Maybe we can finally have that by-God family reunion!

EARL RAY
May as well make yourself at home, Shoff. We're going to be in this shit hole for a while.
          (*grabbing his three
           prosthetic limbs*)
I'm taking a piss today.

BIG AL
You take a piss every day.

EARL RAY
This time I'm standing up. I'm tired of sitting down to piss like a girl. I think I'm ready.

BOBBY MAC
Go for it man.

EARL RAY
          (*wheeling himself behind
           the screen*)
I need you guys nearby. Just in case.

BIG AL
We're right here, Earl, if you need us.

NARRATOR
On the way behind the screen, EARL RAY looks in the mirror next to it. After a moment, he comes back out and looks at the mirror again.

EARL RAY
Told you, Shoff.

JEREMY
I never doubted it, Earl.

EARL RAY
Dumb, fucking shrinks. I'd like to smash that damn thing. I know it was their idea to put a mirror where you have to pass by it to get to the head. No one else would'a done it.

NARRATOR
PAPPY, in a Coast Guard uniform, enters Q ward from stage right. He is carrying a duffel bag in his right hand; his left hand and forearm are covered in white. He looks bewildered and confused.

JEREMY
How's it going?

PAPPY
Doing okay. I'm supposed to bunk here for a couple of weeks. They sent me out here and told me to find an empty bunk. Is this the right place?

BOBBY MAC
Well, hell yeah! Anybody that's got a four-year stripe on his sleeve is welcome on Q! You look like you just seen a fucking ghost! C'mon on in. Grab any bunk as long as it ain't mine.

PAPPY
Thanks. Is anywhere okay?

MOOSE
You got two full legs and both arms, you take a top bunk.

PAPPY
That's not a problem.
          (*putting down his bag, PAPPY
          sits on the stool*)

MOOSE (*pointing*)
Your name tag says Richards. What's your first name?

PAPPY
Sonny.

                    MOOSE
Well, Sonny Richards, what kind of uniform is that you're wearing,
and what are you doing here?

                    PAPPY
               (*looking down at the floor*)
It's Coast Guard. I busted my hand in a training exercise so
they sent me here for a couple of weeks of P.-T.

                    EARL RAY
You're fucking Coast Guard? Jesus Christ, we got us one more noncombat motherfucker. You're in a world of shit. Just ask Shoff.
And if they said you'll be here two weeks, you'll probably be
here a couple of months.

                    PAPPY
Uh, I don't have to bunk here, guys, if it's going to be a problem.

                    BOBBY MAC
Bullshit! We don't really give a shit what you do. You're in
here now and that's that.

                    SKI
Don't dmind Earl. He'll be okay weeth it.

                    PAPPY
You sure it's okay? I can bunk somewhere else.

                    BOBBY MAC
You've come to the right place, my friend. Let me give you a
hand with that duffel bag.

                    PAPPY
Sure, uh, thanks.

                    NARRATOR
BOBBY MAC takes off his rubber hand and tosses it to PAPPY. PAPPY
grabs the hand and stares at it.

                    MOOSE
Give me that damn thing.

                    NARRATOR
MOOSE grabs the hand and the Marines start tossing it back and
forth.

                    EARL RAY
Why the hell did you come through the side doors? You think you
could sneak in here? Maybe steal something?

                    PAPPY
No, not at all. I drove out here from the front gate. They said
go to Q, so I found Q Ward marked on the side of the building and
well, that's where I parked my car.

SKI/JEREMY/BIG AL/MOOSE/ROGER
You what!

PAPPY
Yeah, I drove. My car's sitting right outside.

NARRATOR
BOBBY MAC, JEREMY, SKI, and MOOSE make their ways to stage right and look out, then return to their wheelchairs.

MOOSE
Son of a bitch! Our prayers have been answered.

BOBBY MAC
A genuine by-God limousine if I ever saw one!

BIG AL
Come on in. We've got just the bunk for you!

EARL RAY
A car? So what. Doesn't mean shit. You're letting him in here because he has a car? Another noncombat motherfucker.

PAPPY
Really guys. I can bunk somewhere else.

BOBBY MAC
Not unless you leave us that car, you ain't. Do you know how far it is to the front gate? It takes a guy with both legs twenty minutes.

EARL RAY
(*pointing to JEREMY*)
Yeah, just ask Shoff. Ain't that right noncombat motherfucker.

JEREMY
(*looking straight at EARL RAY*)
Yeah, that's right, Earl. If it makes you feel any better, I'll take a wheelchair the next time and race you to the front.

EARL RAY
(*flexing his right arm muscle*)
Shit, you couldn't beat me with both arms. Remember this?

JEREMY
(*swallowing hard*)
Yeah. I remember it. Don't' get any ideas. I'm never going to hit you, Earl.

EARL RAY
You're still a chicken shit Navy coward.

                                MOOSE
Okay, okay. I thought we left that shit back on 2B. You two
settle this some other time, huh? We'll take a vote. All in
favor of a Coasty staying on Q, raise your hand if you got one.
Otherwise, raise a stump.

                              NARRATOR
Everyone but EARL RAY votes to keep PAPPY on the ward.

                                MOOSE
It's settled. Welcome to Q, Sonny.

                                PAPPY
Thanks guys. I'll try to stay out of the way.

                              EARL RAY
Yeah. Welcome to Q. Just keep your noncombat ass away from me.

                                MOOSE
He'll come around, Sonny. How long have you been in the Coast
Guard?

                                PAPPY
Just over seven years.

                             BOBBY MAC
Shit man, you don't look old enough to be out of high school.

                                PAPPY
Yeah, I'll be twenty-eight my next birthday.

                             BOBBY MAC
No shit! You're an old bastard! By God, we'll just call you
Pappy! Pappy the sailor man.

                               BIG AL
Well, Pappy, you won't mind being our taxi once in a while, will
you?

                                PAPPY
Well, sure. As long as I'm around, I'll take you guys anywhere.

                                MOOSE
Perfect, Pappy, this bunk right over here is yours. Welcome to
Q.

                                 SKI
Djust another beautiful day in paradise!

                             BOBBY MAC
Sure as hell beats Nam.

                              EARL RAY
Yeah, well, it was Nam that put us in this shithole.

MOOSE
This ain't so bad, Earl. It won't be long before we all get out of here and head home.

EARL RAY
What the fuck is home? I'm never going home. Ain't shit in Florida anymore.

SKI
Are you steel getting letters from Jendeefer?

EARL RAY
Yeah, I'm still getting letters from <u>Jendeefer</u>.

SKI
dWhat does she have to say?

EARL RAY
How the hell would I know? I haven't read any of them.

SKI
dWhat the hell do dyou do weeth them, Earl?

EARL RAY
I just toss 'em in my locker.

MOOSE
They're in your locker? Unopened?

EARL RAY
That's what I said, didn't I?

SKI
dYou are a lucky guy, Earl. dYou should read them. dYou should call her someday.

EARL RAY
Yeah, like I said before. Maybe someday when I'm feeling lucky.

MOOSE
That day will come, Earl. The day you get out of here will be your lucky day. None of us can stay in here forever.

EARL RAY
Maybe I won't make it out of here. Maybe I don't want to.

MOOSE
C'mon, Earl, that's no way to talk.

EARL RAY
The way I see it, I've got two choices. Live the rest of my life stuck in this fucking chair, or finish what the land mine didn't do.

                    MOOSE
Shit, Earl, you can come live with me.

                    EARL RAY
You're really funny, Moose.

                    MOOSE
I'm not being funny, my friend. Think about it, will you?

                    EARL RAY
Yeah. I'll think about it. Got nowhere else to go.

                    MOOSE
             (looking at SKI)
Hey, Ski, how's that new plastic leg fitting you?

                    SKI (grinning)
Like a glove.

                    BOBBY MAC
Shit. If your leg fits like a glove, then my hand fits like a shoe!

          Everyone laughs.

                    MOOSE
How about you, Big Al? You're standing tall in that rocking horse you use sometimes, my friend.

                    BIG AL
Giddy up! I'm ready to ride.

                    JEREMY
That sounds like a plan. Tell you what, Big Al, how about you and me go out and find a place to have a few beers?

                    BIG AL
Yeah, you and me, and this anchor on my ass.

                    JEREMY
You don't need that rocking horse, you got me.

                    BIG AL
What do you mean?

                    JEREMY
Just what I said. Get off that high horse of yours and let's go.

                    NARRATOR
JEREMY bends down. BIG AL grabs JEREMY around the neck. JEREMY stands up, lifting BIG AL onto his back. BIG AL is smiling from ear to ear.

JEREMY
Climb on, Big Al. We're going places!

*JEREMY and BIG AL head
toward the side door.*

JEREMY
We'll head north to the first street and take a look around.
This is a Navy base. There has to be a bar nearby.

BIG AL
I go where you go.

*JEREMY and BIG AL exit
stage right.*

BIG AL (O.S.)
Oh, look! There one is, Shoff! The Rainbow Bar and Grille.

JEREMY (O.S.)
Hell of a name for a bar, ain't it?

BIG AL (O.S.)
Doesn't matter to me if they <u>name</u> it Hell. Just get me inside!

JEREMY and BIG AL laugh.

*Lights fade and go out,
one at a time, stage right
to stage left.*

ACT II

SCENE 2

SETTING: *FOR NINE-ACTOR READERS THEATER CASTING AND SEATING CHART, SEE PAGE 3. For both acts, all scenes: nine seats are in a row from left to right. If six wheelchairs are available, they should be used for seats 1,2,3 and 7,8,9. The center three seats (4,5,6) should be chairs or stools. The NARRATOR sits off the stage, at either side. In front of each seat is a stand holding a copy of the script.*

If costumes are available, during the second act MOOSE, BIG AL, EARL RAY, SKI, and BOBBY MAC wear USMC uniforms. JEREMY wears a US Navy uniform; PAPPY (in seat 4) wears a US Coast Guard uniform. EVA (seat 5) wears a silky robe over her hotpants. BAR PATRON (seat 6) wears a puffy, insulated vest over his dark pants and an open necked shirt.

AT RISE: *From stage left to stage right, seated are: MOOSE, BIG AL, EARL RAY, PAPPY, EVA, BAR PATRON, SKI, JEREMY, BOBBY MAC.*

NARRATOR
Three bar-height tables with three chairs at each one are arranged left to right at the Rainbow Bar and Grill. JEREMY and BIG AL sit at the table to the audience's left. EVA and one of her regular BAR PATRONs are sitting at the table on the right. As the lights come up on each seat in order, the BAR PATRON is carrying JEREMY and BIG AL a pitcher of beer and two glasses on a tray.

BAR PATRON
Let me get these for you.

JEREMY/BIG AL
Thanks, man! We sure appreciate it.

NARRATOR
BAR PATRON sits with EVA at the table stage left. They talk quietly for a moment as JEREMY and BIG AL drink and BAR PATRON nods his head towards JEREMY and BIG AL. EVA gets up and dances her way over to sit down next to BIG AL. She flicks a finger nail at the hospital band on BIG AL's left wrist and holds BIG AL by the hand.

EVA
Nice to have you guys here. What're your names?

BIG AL
(*a little nervous*)
I'm Al. Big Al. Everyone calls me Big Al. This is Shoff.

                                EVA
                    (*glancing at where BIG AL's
                    legs should be*)
Nice to know you. Not many guys from over there come in here.
Did you two walk all the way here? I mean, did you come all the
way from the front? That's a long way to --

                              BIG AL
It's okay. We took a short cut. Actually, we made us a short cut
through a hole in the fence.

                              JEREMY
It's really not that far. We're glad we found this place.

                                EVA
                    (*tapping BIG AL's patient
                    ID bracelet*)
Let's see, Shoff. You wearing one of these patient IDs, too?

                              JEREMY
Yeah.

                                EVA
                    (*getting up to go back to
                    her bar stool*)
You two enjoy yourselves. Come in anytime and bring your friends
if you want. This is my bar and it's open to you anytime.

                             NARRATOR
BAR PATRON brings over another pitcher of beer.

                              JEREMY
I think we should call the others, Big Al. How about you?

                              BIG AL
                    (*looking at EVA*)
Yeah. I think that's a really good idea.

                              JEREMY
                    (*to Eva*)
Thanks, Eva, for that gracious invitation, and thanks, everyone,
for the beer! Would you keep Big Al company for a few minutes,
Eva? I'm going to call a few of our friends and tell them about
this great place we've found.

                    *JEREMY walks behind the
                    screen and you can hear
                    his voice offstage.*

                           JEREMY (O.S.)
Hey, Earl Ray! We found a place just around the corner. Just
turn north when you come out the side doors. The Rainbow Bar and
Grille. Nice lady over here. Ya'll come quick. It's nice.
                              (MORE)

         JEREMY (O.S.) (CONT'D)
Real nice.
         (walking back to the table)
Any minute now. They'll be here any minute.

                    NARRATOR
JEREMY and BIG AL drink beer until EARL RAY, MOOSE, BOBBY MAC and
SKI come out from behind the screen.

                    BIG AL
What took you so long?

                    JEREMY
Yeah. We got tired of waiting. Where's Pappy?

                    MOOSE
He's parking the car. If Earl doesn't like it here, he's ready
to take him back.

                    NARRATOR
PAPPY comes in and sits with them.

                    BIG AL
That was quick!

                    PAPPY
I sure don't want to miss out on a good thing.

                    EVA
Good to see you men. Let's see if we can fix you guys up.

                    NARRATOR
EVA and BAR PATRON help move the two tables stage right and center
together and move the empty stools to those tables, making seven
stools at the joined tables and only two stools at the table stage
left. EVA sits at the table stage left and nods to BAR PATRON.

                    BAR PATRON
Looks like you men need another pitcher.

                    NARRATOR
BAR PATRON carries over another pitcher and five more glasses,
then joins EVA at their table.

                    EARL RAY
The Rainbow. That's a hell-of-a-name for a bar.

                    BIG AL
Like I told Shoff, they could call it Hell for all I care. It's
real close to the hospital, they got cold beer, and Eva is my
kind of woman.

                    EARL RAY
Any woman is your kind of woman.

BIG AL
Not the kind of woman you're thinking of. She gives a shit.

EARL RAY
Ain't no woman gives a shit.

BIG AL
Why don't you find out for yourself?

EARL RAY
Yeah, right. Like some broad you met at a bar is going to give a shit about me.

BIG AL
She ain't some broad. If you got out once in a while, you'd see they ain't all broads.

EARL RAY
Why did she take a liking to your ass? It ain't like you got one.

BIG AL
She's just that way. Ain't that right, Shoff?

JEREMY
First woman I've ever known that gives a shit. She's real, Earl. She owns the place. Came right over to us and sat down next to Big Al.

BIG AL
She's a good dancer, too.

SKI
Her dname is Eva and she dances, too?

BIG AL
That's right, smart ass. And she bought us each a pitcher of beer.

EARL RAY
Remember. If I don't like it here, we ain't staying. Got it?

MOOSE
Got it, Earl.

BIG AL
Can we get four pitchers down here real quick?

EVA
No time to even say hello? What's the hurry? And why wouldn't you like it here? Did these two tell you what a witch I am? The name's Eva. And you are?

                    EARL RAY
Earl Ray.

                    EVA
Well, Earl Ray, you have a handsome face and wonderful blue eyes. And your names?

                    NARRATOR
Each patient in turn says his name out loud.

                    EVA
Nice to meet all of you. I'll be back to check on you in a bit.

                    NARRATOR
EVA returns to the stage left table and nods at BAR PATRON to deliver four more pitchers of beer.

                    BIG AL
I told you she gives a shit.

                    EARL RAY
We've been here two minutes.

                    BIG AL
That's all you need.

                    MOOSE
What do you think, Earl? You want to stay awhile?

                    EARL RAY (*shrugging*)
Got nothing else to do.

                    JEREMY
Anybody need anything?

                    EARL RAY
Yeah. I want to see if that broad dances as good as Big Al says she does.

                    BIG AL
She ain't a broad, Earl.

                    MOOSE
Okay, okay. Shoff, go see if she can settle this, will you?

                    NARRATOR
JEREMY walks over to EVA.

                    EVA
What's up, Shoff?

                    JEREMY
Earl Ray swears you can't dance.

EVA
Is that so? Seems Earl Ray needs a little personal attention. Does he have any particular song in mind? Or is it my choice?

JEREMY
I think he would be glad if you did the honors.

NARRATOR
EVA moves behind the screen.

BIG AL
You must have scared the little lady.

EARL RAY
I knew she didn't give a shit.

BIG AL
Yeah, we'll see.

JEREMY
I think I could spend a lot of time here.

BOBBY MAC
You got that right. Shit, it may be just a little too close. Look there, Shoff.

NARRATOR
EVA, who has added a slinky dress over her hotpants, dances gracefully from behind the screen to EARL RAY, never taking her eyes off him.

EVA
Just you and me, Earl.
         (*gently kissing EARL RAY*)
Just you and me.
         (*caressing EARL RAY's face*)
You are the bravest man I have ever met.

BIG AL
I told you so!

        Lights fade and go out,
        one at a time, stage right
        to stage left.

ACT II

SCENE 3

SETTING: *FOR NINE-ACTOR READERS THEATER CASTING AND SEATING CHART, SEE PAGE 3. For both acts, all scenes: nine seats are in a row from left to right. If six wheelchairs are available, they should be used for seats 1,2,3 and 7,8,9. The center three seats (4,5,6) should be chairs or stools. The NARRATOR sits off the stage, at either side. In front of each seat is a stand holding a copy of the script.*

If costumes are available, JEREMY is wearing his US Navy everyday white uniform and BIG AL is wearing his USMC non-dress khaki uniform. ROSIE is wearing a skirt split all the way to her crotch.

AT RISE: *From stage left to stage right, seated are: an empty wheelchair, BIG AL, and an empty wheelchair; an empty stool, ROSIE and another empty stool; and an empty, JEREMY, and an empty wheelchairs.*

NARRATOR
As the lights come up, JEREMY and BIG AL are sitting on a bus bench in front of an old home covered with pink and purple gingerbread ornaments. The yard is surrounded by a decorative cast iron fence. It is classic. Tasteful. Inviting. JEREMY has been carrying BIG AL on his back, and the two are resting.

JEREMY
Man, I can't believe Pappy was deployed back to his duty station in Florida when he only had five months left. How're we ever going to get Earl Ray out of the hospital again?

BIG AL
I don't know. And just about the time I thought you and Pappy would finally prove Earl Ray wrong.

JEREMY
You mean about who we are? Well, <u>you</u> might have thought he'd change his mind about our being noncombat motherfuckers, but <u>I</u> don't think he ever will. Pappy and I will be noncombat motherfuckers to Earl till the day we die. Pass me that pack, will you?

BIG AL
(*passing JEREMY a pack of cigarettes*)
It would have helped if he could have sold Earl that old Buick.

JEREMY
Yeah. That would have helped us get Earl back and forth to the Rainbow, for sure, but it was Pappy's only way to get back to his duty station in Florida. That car is all he had.

JEREMY
Well, until he gets out. He might come back. Five months, he said.

BIG AL
Who knows? Maybe he'll come back after that.

NARRATOR
JEREMY pulls two cigarettes from the pack, lights them, smokes one and hands the other one to BIG AL.

BIG AL
Thanks, my friend.

NARRATOR
ROSIE, who has been watching BIG AL and JEREMY sitting on their bus stop bench from inside her house, gets up out of her chair and approaches them.

ROSIE
You two going to sit here all day?

BIG AL
Not me. It's hurting my ass.

ROSIE
The name's Rosie, nice to meet you two.

BIG AL
I'm Big Al, this here's Shoff.

ROSIE
Well, Big Al and Shoff, what brings you to my bus stop? My friends and I have been watching you for almost half an hour.

BIG AL
Just resting a while. This walking takes a lot out of me.

ROSIE
I'm sure it does. Why don't you two come in and have a beer?

JEREMY/BIG AL
Are you kidding me? Sure!

NARRATOR
ROSIE and JEREMY, with BIG AL around his neck, cross the stage to enter her living room. It has padded purple and lavender chairs with a matching couch, a coffee table with a rotary dial phone on it, a lamp with a fringed shade, and at the back, a doorway with a beaded hanging screen revealing a glimpse of an unseen room.

ROSIE
You two make yourselves comfortable. I'll get us something to drink.

NARRATOR
ROSIE goes behind the screen while BIG AL and JEREMY sit and look around.

                    JEREMY
              (*excited and nervous*)
You thinking what I'm thinking?

                    BIG AL
              (*excited*)
Yeah, Rosie runs a whore house! Somebody pinch me.

                    JEREMY
Of all the bus benches we could have picked. Damn good thing my
legs were getting tired when they did.

                    BIG AL
Don't you dare take all the credit. Shit, it was my idea to give
you a rest. I don't think we have enough money for this place.

                    JEREMY
That's for damn sure.

                    NARRATOR
ROSIE comes back in with two mugs of beer and three glasses of
wine on a tray.

                    BIG AL
Wow, you really like your wine. And only one beer for us?

                    ROSIE
These are for my friends upstairs. Hope you like Budweiser.

                    NARRATOR
Laughing, Rosie puts the beer and one glass of wine on the table,
then takes the other two wines offstage.

                    JEREMY (*grinning*)
Did you hear that, Big Al? She has two friends upstairs!

                    BIG AL
              (*tips his beer towards JEREMY*)
The King of Beers.

                    NARRATOR
As ROSIE comes back in, BIG AL squirms on his chair.

                    ROSIE
Would you be more comfortable sitting here, Al?

                    BIG AL
I'm okay. I'm just not used to nice pillows. The ones we have
on Q are like bricks.

                    ROSIE
What's Q?

BIG AL
Oh, sorry. It's the ward we live on at the Navy hospital. Q ward.

ROSIE
(*raising her glass to toast*)
Well, here's to Q ward. And, I prefer to call this a Garden of Eden. Don't let Tammie and Sheryl hear you call it a whore house.

BIG AL
Sorry, we didn't mean anything by it. But you do -- you are -- I mean --

ROSIE
Yes, we do, and yes, we are. But we are very much ladies. And we don't walk the streets or hustle the bars.

JEREMY
Then how do you, you know.

ROSIE
We refer to them as clients, and they know how to find us. But this time we found you. Now, how do we get you upstairs, Big Al?

JEREMY
That's my job.

BIG AL
Can you believe this?

NARRATOR
JEREMY carries BIG AL behind the screen and returns to the couch without him.

ROSIE
What about you, um, Shoff? Would you like to meet Sheryl?

JEREMY
I think I'll just wait for Big Al. You know we don't have a lot of mon --

ROSIE
Please, don't. You and your friend are our guests. We invited you here. We are doing this because we want to. Sure you don't want to meet Sheryl?

JEREMY
(*sitting on the couch*)
I'll just wait for Big Al.

ROSIE
(*sits next to JEREMY on the couch*)
She'll be more than disappointed. Are you trying to be noble?

JEREMY
No. I don't think I even know how to be. I just want this to be something special for Big Al.

ROSIE
What would Al say about you saying no?

JEREMY
He's going to think I'm nuts. He'll recommend me for the psych ward.

ROSIE
You can still change your mind.

JEREMY
Maybe next time. I mean if --

ROSIE
Of course, there will be a next time. You and Al are welcome anytime. Well, almost any time. We'll have to set up some rules. Let me think about it. I really don't like calling you Shoff. Do you have a first name?

JEREMY
Jeremy.

ROSIE
Well, Jeremy, what brought you two to my front gate?

JEREMY
Well, the Rainbow isn't the same without Earl Ray, so we were looking for a new place.

ROSIE
The Rainbow?

JEREMY
Yeah, the Rainbow. It's a bar close to the hospital.

ROSIE
And Earl Ray?

JEREMY
A friend of mine and Big Al's. A best friend.

ROSIE
He must be if you don't want to go to the Rainbow without him.

JEREMY
It's the only way we can get him out of the hospital. He lost both of his legs and his left arm in Viet Nam. The Rainbow is a special place for Earl Ray. It's where he can sit and talk with Eva. Sometimes they sit and talk for a couple of hours.

ROSIE

Who is Eva?

JEREMY

She owns the Rainbow. She's the only woman Earl Ray will talk to, well, except for Jennifer. And now, he doesn't talk to her very often.

ROSIE

Who's Jennifer?

JEREMY

Earl Ray's fiancé. She sends him letters every week. He just puts them in his locker unopened. Must be thirty or forty of them.

ROSIE

Why can't you get Earl Ray back over to the Rainbow?

JEREMY

Well, it's a long story. But mostly because Pappy left with his Buick and without his legs, Earl Ray doesn't have a way to get around.

ROSIE

I know that must make sense to you, Jeremy. But who's Pappy and what happened to him?

JEREMY

Pappy was another patient on Q. His ancient Buick was the only way to get Earl Ray over to the Rainbow. But then Pappy was sent back to full duty and Earl Ray hasn't left Q ward ever since.

ROSIE

It sounds like Earl Ray could use some personal attention. Maybe you can bring him by. Or maybe one of us could pick you guys up sometime. We'll talk about it.

JEREMY

That would be great if we could get him to come.

BIG AL (O.S.)
(*singing*)
Oh, Jeremy! I'm do-one! Come get me!

NARRATOR

JEREMY goes behind the screen and comes back with BIG AL, who he helps into one of the chairs.

BIG AL

Oh, Jeremy! I think I'm in love! Tammie was magic.

ROSIE

You should see your cheeks, Al. Now you know why it's called Rosie's Place.
    (to JEREMY)
See what you missed, Jeremy?

JEREMY

Man, I'm going to recommend myself to the psych ward.

BIG AL

What do mean? Didn't you? You what?

ROSIE

That's right, Al. He didn't.

BIG AL

You gotta be shitting me!

ROSIE

It's okay, Jeremy. Maybe next time? Speaking of next time. I've thought about the rules. This is our secret; you tell anyone other than Earl Ray and it's off. No more than once a week. After all, it is a business. Call the number I gave you before you want to come down. Friday and Sunday afternoons are best. Sit on the bus bench until one of us comes out. Oh, and don't forget to talk to Earl Ray.
    (kissing BIG AL and JEREMY
     on their cheeks)
And remember, we are ladies here.

JEREMY/BIG AL

Wow! Thank you, Rosie! Thanks for everything!

NARRATOR

JEREMY carries BIG AL back to the bench and sits next to him. They light cigarettes and smoke.

BIG AL

I think I'm in love, Shoff.

JEREMY

I don't blame you, Al.

BIG AL

No, I mean it. I think I'm in love. I could feel it. She held me like a baby. I mean, she didn't just screw me, she made love to me. I don't think I've ever had a woman do that before.

JEREMY

Be careful, Al, that's what she does for a living. Tammie may not even be her real name.

                              BIG AL
I don't give a shit. I've never felt like that with a woman
before.

                              JEREMY
Maybe it's the kind of women you've been with before.

                              BIG AL
She's different, man. I know she's supposed to make you feel
good, but I'll bet other guys don't feel like this about her.
Shit, they all probably got wives at home.

                              JEREMY
Let's talk about it back on Q.

                              BIG AL
No, I just want to sit here a while.

                              JEREMY
Okay with me. We've got all night.

                JEREMY and BIG AL sit in
                silence for a moment.

                              BIG AL
I don't want to go back to Q.

                              JEREMY
We got to go in some time. People are going to wonder about us
after a while.

                              BIG AL
No, Shoff, I really don't want to go back inside there.

                              JEREMY
Okay, Al. Whatever you want. We can sit here the rest of our
lives if you want to.

                              BIG AL
I wish she hadn't been so nice to me. Ain't no way I'm going to
meet another woman that can make me feel like she did.

                              JEREMY
I think there's women out there, Al. It just takes what it took
tonight to find them.

                              BIG AL
Yeah, what's that?

                              JEREMY
Pure fucking luck.

II-3-74

                    BIG AL
Yeah, maybe you're right. Maybe it is pure fucking luck.
                    (*pause*)
C'mon, Shoff. Get me inside. I gotta piss.

           JEREMY laughs.

               The lights fade out, one
               at a time, stage right to
               stage left.

ACT II

SCENE 4

SETTING: *FOR NINE-ACTOR READERS THEATER CASTING AND SEATING CHART, SEE PAGE 3. For both acts, all scenes: nine seats are in a row from left to right. If six wheelchairs are available, they should be used for seats 1,2,3 and 7,8,9. The center three seats (4,5,6) should be chairs or stools. The NARRATOR sits off the stage, at either side. In front of each seat is a stand holding a copy of the script.*

If costumes are available, JEREMY is wearing his US Navy everyday white uniform and BIG AL is wearing his USMC non-dress khaki uniform. ROSIE is wearing a skirt split all the way to her crotch.

AT RISE: *From stage left to stage right, seated are: an empty wheelchair, BIG AL, and an empty wheelchair; an empty stool, ROSIE and another empty stool; an empty wheelchair, JEREMY, and another empty wheelchair.*

NARRATOR
As the lights come up, JEREMY walks to the rear of the left side of the stage, where there is a rotary-dial phone on a small table. He dials a number from a piece of paper he pulls out of his pocket. As he is making his phone call, ROSIE gets up from where she is sitting in a large padded chair on the right side of the stage. Her living room has padded purple and lavender chairs with a matching couch, a coffee table with a rotary dial phone on it, a lamp with a fringed shade, and at the back, a doorway with a beaded hanging screen revealing a glimpse of an unseen room. She answers the phone.

ROSIE
(*into phone*)
Hello. This is Rosie.

JEREMY
(*into phone*)
Hi Rosie, it's Shoff.

ROSIE
(*into phone*)
Hi Jeremy. How have you been? I thought I would have heard from you sooner than this. Have you and Al forgotten about me?

JEREMY
(*into phone*)
Not hardly, Rosie. We've talked about you, Tammie, and Sheryl every day. Just me and Big Al that is. Well, and Earl Ray.

ROSIE
(*into phone*)
And what does Earl Ray think?

JEREMY
(*into phone*)
Just like Earl. At first, he said it was bullshit. The more we told him about it, the more he's convinced Big Al had a religious experience.

ROSIE
(*into phone*)
That's too funny.

JEREMY
(*into phone*)
Not for Big Al. He thinks he's in love with Tammie. He thinks if he stays away, he can forget about her.

ROSIE
(*into phone*)
And what do you think, Jeremy?

JEREMY
(*into phone*)
What do I think? Well, I think in his mind, he is in love with Tammie.

ROSIE
(*into phone*)
And does that bother you?

JEREMY
(*into phone*)
What would bother me is if Big Al gets screwed. I mean screwed over.

ROSIE
(*into phone*)
Trust me. Tammie knows what she's doing. She wants to see Al again.

JEREMY
(*into phone*)
Hold on a second. I want you to tell him what you just told me.

NARRATOR
JEREMY carries BIG Al the phone.

BIG AL
(*into phone*)
Rosie? Big Al. How's it hangin'?

ROSIE
(*into phone*)
Just fine, Al. Listen, this is a pretty good time for us. Why don't you and Jeremy come on over? Tammie wants to see you.

NARRATOR
BIG AL turns 360 degrees in his wheelchair.

BIG AL
Shoff, I told you so!

JEREMY
(*into phone*)
Rosie?

ROSIE
(*into phone*)
Come on over, okay?

JEREMY
(*into phone*)
We're on our way.

NARRATOR
JEREMY picks up BIG AL and carries him across the stage, through ROSIE's living room, to behind the screen. ROSIE follows them. When they come back out, JEREMY is carrying BIG AL on his back, but is wearing only his uniform trousers and a tee shirt. ROSIE is carrying JEREMY's uniform shirt. JEREMY puts BIG AL in one of the chairs, and JEREMY and ROSIE sit on the couch.

ROSIE
That was nice. We'll have to do this again sometime.

JEREMY
That would be nice, Rosie.

ROSIE
You two look ecstatic. Would you like something to drink?

JEREMY
A couple of beers would be great. Thanks, Rosie.

ROSIE
Nice to see everyone smiling. Must have been a good afternoon.

JEREMY
The only thing better would have been Earl Ray with us.

BIG AL
Yeah. If we could only get him here.

ROSIE
I've heard a lot about Earl Ray. When do you think I can meet him?

JEREMY
We're not sure Earl Ray wants to go anywhere. Sometimes he thinks he's a pain in the ass to everybody, including himself.

BIG AL
Shit, we'd take him anywhere he wants. We'd do anything for him. He just doesn't see it that way. Besides, I think it's mostly Jennifer.

ROSIE
From what you've told me, Jeremy, Jennifer's his whole life. Or used to be. Tell you what. If you can get Earl Ray to say yes to me, I'm sure Sheryl would be more than happy to come pick him up.

BIG AL
It's worth a try. He needs to get out before he goes nuts or drives us nuts.

JEREMY
He needs to get out before he does something we'll all regret.

ROSIE
What do you mean by that, Jeremy?

JEREMY
We promised him he could choose to end his life. If that's what he wants. We promised we wouldn't stop him.

ROSIE
Then let's get him over here and see if we can convince him he doesn't want to do that.

*Lights fade and go out,
one at a time, stage right
to stage left.*

ACT II

SCENE 5

SETTING: *FOR NINE-ACTOR READERS THEATER CASTING AND SEATING CHART, SEE PAGE 3. For both acts, all scenes: nine seats are in a row from left to right. If six wheelchairs are available, they should be used for seats 1,2,3 and 7,8,9. The center three seats (4,5,6) should be chairs or stools. The NARRATOR sits off the stage, at either side. In front of each seat is a stand holding a copy of the script.*

If costumes are available, JEREMY is wearing his US Navy everyday white uniform and EARL RAY and BIG AL are wearing USMC non-dress khaki uniforms. ROSIE is wearing a skirt split all the way up the middle to her crotch.

AT RISE: *From stage left to stage right, seated are: an empty wheelchair, BIG AL and EARL RAY in wheelchairs; an empty stool, ROSIE and another empty stool; and an empty, JEREMY, and an empty wheelchairs.*

NARRATOR
JEREMY, carrying BIG AL on his back and pushing EARL RAY's wheelchair, follows ROSIE into her living room. EARL RAY is carrying crutches. ROSIE is wearing a skirt split up the middle all the way up to her crotch. With BIG AL still on his back, JEREMY parks EARL RAY's chair next to Rosie's.

ROSIE
Tammie is waiting and time is wasting, don't you think, Al?

BIG AL
We'll see you guys in a couple of hours. Don't do anything I wouldn't do!

NARRATOR
JEREMY carries BIG AL behind the screen.

ROSIE
We're so glad you decided to come, Earl. We've heard a lot about you. You have two very special friends.

EARL RAY
Big Al, maybe. I'm not sure I would call Shoff special.

JEREMY comes back out and sits on the couch.

JEREMY
You'll never get a Marine to call anyone in the Navy special.

EARL RAY
Got that right, noncombat -- I won't say that in front of the ladies.

                    ROSIE
Thank you, Earl for calling us ladies. We love you already.

                    ROSIE
What about you, Earl? Sheryl would like to get to know you.
          (*pointing towards screen*)
If you'd like to get to meet her, she's right through there.

                    EARL RAY
I don't know. Maybe some other time.

                    ROSIE
It's okay. You can just talk if you want. She won't do anything
you don't want to do.

                    EARL RAY
Okay. I'll give it a try. Just get me in there, Shoff, then get
out.

                    NARRATOR
JEREMY pushes EARL RAY behind the purple screen, with ROSIE
following.

                    EARL RAY (O.S.)
Give me my crutches, Shoff! I can do this myself!

                    JEREMY (O.S.)
Get one under his right arm, Rosie!

                    ROSIE (O.S.)
Got it, Jeremy. You're okay, Earl.

                    EARL RAY (O.S.)
I'm okay. Just wasn't watching where I was going. Now, get out
of here, Shoff! I don't need your fucking help!

                    NARRATOR
ROSIE and JEREMY return to the living room and sit on the couch.

                    EARL RAY (O.S.)
Told you, Shoff!

                    JEREMY
I never doubted it, Earl.

                    ROSIE
He means a lot to you, doesn't he, Jeremy?

                    JEREMY
He's my hero, Rosie. And you know what? He's never asked for a
fucking thing. Not one god damn thing. He's more of a man than
I'll ever be. And don't dare pity him. He'll kill you if you
do. Don't let him see you give a shit, either.
                    (MORE)

                          JEREMY (CONT'D)
No, don't do that. That means he has to give a shit back. That's
the way he is. There's only so much loyalty for him to give, but
when he does give it to you, it matters. It means something.
Ask Ski and Moose and Big Al. Ask any Marine. Ask Jennifer.
I'll never earn it. I've tried. I don't deserve it. He tried
to kill me once. He could have, too, but I believe he really
didn't want to. He's accepted me, but he'll never trust me. He
pushes back on every fucking thing. He pisses me off, but I think
he knows I love him like a brother. He deserves more than any of
us can ever give him, but he'll never take anything from anyone
he doesn't trust. Don't ever owe anybody anything. That's Earl --
and he's never once asked for a god damn thing.

                              ROSIE
C'mon Jeremy, let's go upstairs.

                            NARRATOR
ROSIE takes JEREMY by the hand and leads him behind the screen.
After a few moments, voices are heard from off stage.

                          FEMALE VOICE (O.S.)
Help me! Someone help! Please hurry!

                          JEREMY (O.S.)
Holy shit! He's having a flashback! He might be killing her!

                          BIG AL (O.S.)
Get me in there, Shoff! Quick! Hurry, Shoff!

                          JEREMY (O.S.)
We're coming, Earl. Hold on, Earl. Just hold on.

                          FEMALE VOICE (O.S.)
I'm okay. Really. It's just that my pubic hairs are stuck in
his legs. Please help me get them out. As fast as you can.

                          BIG AL (O.S.)
Oh, wow! Just hold really still, okay Earl? We can fix this.

                          EARL RAY (O.S.)
Get me out of here. Get me back to Q.

                          FEMALE VOICE (O.S.)
It's okay, Earl. What if we take them off? I'll be okay, I think.

                          EARL RAY (O.S.)
Just get me out of here and get me back to Q.

                          ROSIE (O.S.)
Maybe we can sit in the living room for a while.

                          JEREMY (O.S.)
What do you think, Al?

                        BIG AL (O.S.)
        Just get me back to Q, Shoff. Get us back to Q.

                    *Lights fade out and turn
                    off, one at a time, stage
                    right to stage left.*

ACT II

SCENE 6

SETTING: *FOR NINE-ACTOR READERS THEATER CASTING AND SEATING CHART, SEE PAGE 3. For both acts, all scenes: nine seats are in a row from left to right. If six wheelchairs are available, they should be used for seats 1,2,3 and 7,8,9. The center three seats (4,5,6) should be chairs or stools. The NARRATOR sits off the stage, at either side. In front of each seat is a stand holding a copy of the script.*

If costumes are available, MOOSE, BIG AL, EARL RAY, SKI, and BOBBY MAC wear USMC uniforms. JEREMY and TINY wear US Navy uniforms. SGT. PEPPER and HIPPIE are dressed as hippies.

AT RISE: *From stage left to stage right, seated are: MOOSE, BIG AL, and EARL RAY, in wheelchairs; TINY, HIPPIE, and SGT. PEPPER, on the stools; and SKI, JEREMY, and BOBBY MAC, in wheelchairs.*

NARRATOR
As the lights come up, BOBBY MAC, JEREMY, SKI, EARL RAY, BIG AL, and MOOSE are in the wheelchairs, set up as the rows in a bus, all facing in the same direction. TINY is in the driver's seat at the head of the bus, addressing JEREMY.

TINY
Jeremy, it's been my pleasure to have you work for me in Special Services these past few months. Today's trip is the last one of the summer, and, as you know, it is indeed special.

JEREMY
Thanks, Tiny. It's been fun, and you helped make it that way. I think I can speak for everybody here, this trip to Atlantic City for the weekend is something we all thank you for. We know how lucky we are to have been picked for this trip.

TINY
You're lucky <u>any</u> of you were <u>ever</u> picked for another trip after that last clam bake!

JEREMY
Well, if the band hadn't played "Mr. Lonely" and dedicated "Coming Home Soldier" to -- and I quote -- "their special audience," all of those emotions wouldn't have swept through the festivities like a fire through a funeral pyre. But, oh, my God, wasn't it a great ending to the day? Corn cobs, chicken bones, clam shells, and paper plates flying everywhere? Tables and wheelchairs and plastic and wooden body parts all over the place, and people hiding under the tables and tablecloths? God, it was <u>great</u>. I think the only thing not being thrown was the beer, and that's only because we were drinking it as fast as we could.

                    TINY (*laughing*)
Okay, well, that was pretty spectacular. And then for it to stop,
all of a sudden, with everyone laughing, shaking hands, and
embracing? It was, I admit, one of the coolest things I've ever
seen. And just so you know, when I asked "What are you going to
do for an encore," that didn't mean you should repeat the
performance this weekend.

                         JEREMY
Wouldn't think of it, Tiny. We'll be on our best behavior. I
promise.

                        NARRATOR
JEREMY and TINY enter "the bus," TINY standing at the front, facing
the wheelchairs, and JEREMY going to the back.

                          TINY
So, who's gonna win?
              (*confused looks from the
               others*)
Miss America, you bums! That's why we're going to Atlantic City
for crying out loud.

                     JEREMY/SKI/MOOSE
Oh!

                         MOOSE
I don't even know who's in the contest.

                          TINY
For God's sake. Just name a state!

                        EARL RAY
Shit, Moose, you ever hear of Miss America before today?

                       BOBBY MAC
You got fifty chances. Go for it.

                        BIG AL
I don't care who wins. Ain't none of them can come close to Tammie.

                       EARL RAY
I still don't know why she's taken a liking to your ass.

                        BIG AL
What's it matter, Earl? She'S a lot like Jennifer, you know.

                       EARL RAY
What do you know about it?

                        BIG AL
I know Jennifer would give her life for you. Shit, man. Wake up
before it's too late.

> EARL RAY
> (*raising his prosthetic arm
> and hook into the air*)

Look at me. It's already too late.

> SKI

Eets never too late. Dyou should read Jendeefer's letters. How the hell dyou know if eets too late.

> EARL RAY

'Cause I said so. Maybe I don't want to know what is in those letters.

> BOBBY MAC

You keep them for a reason, my friend.

> EARL RAY
> (*staring out the window*)

Well, it's none of your business.

> MOOSE

You're one of us, Earl. That makes it our business.

> EARL RAY
> (*reaching in shirt pocket*)

The only thing that would help right now is another pain pill, and for you guys to shut up about it.

> MOOSE

Okay, Earl. We'll give it a break for now. Just be careful with those things. You scared the shit out of us the last time you took too many.

> EARL RAY

You can never take too many.

> BOBBY MAC

Got to take it easy with that shit, Earl. We need you around to keep us in line. We all need some of it, but take it easy.

> EARL RAY

Just back off for now.

> TINY
> (*putting a hand on EARL
> RAY's shoulder*)

They're right, Earl. You and I have talked about this before. I should have reported it the last time, but God help me, I didn't. I can't keep turning a blind eye.

> EARL RAY

I'm okay, Tiny. I'm okay.

TINY
We better get going. It's four hours to the hotel and they have a Friday night all-you-can-eat buffet waiting for us.

SKI
WoooHooo! Follow dthe yellow brick droad!

NARRATOR
TINY and JEREMY sit in their seats. A female HIPPIE wearing hippie clothes and SGT. PEPPER, a long-haired male in his early twenties wearing Marine corps fatigues, both adorned with peace emblem headbands, hippie hats and leather fringe vests, enter the stage from stage left and step in front of the bus.

HIPPIE
(*flipping them the finger*)
Hey, fuck you, baby killers!

SGT. PEPPER
I'm ashamed of what I did in Nam, and you should be, too!

MOOSE
Fuck you, you long-haired motherfucker! Stay right there and I'll baby-kill your ass!

BOBBY MAC
Yeah, you chicken-shit asshole!

SGT. PEPPER
(*giving the finger*)
Fuck you, man! You baby-killing bastards!

NARRATOR
As HIPPIE stands in front of bus, SGT. PEPPER moves to beside EARL RAY.

EARL RAY
(*hitting in SGT. PEPPER's direction*)
How 'bout this, motherfucker!

SGT. PEPPER
Shit! What the fuck! I'll kill <u>your</u> ass.

NARRATOR
TINY, MOOSE and JEREMY jump off the bus and start pounding on SGT. PEPPER.

TINY
Okay, asshole. Who's next?

HIPPIE
Get off him! Get off him!

TINY
(*grabbing MOOSE's shoulder*)
Okay, Moose. He's had enough. Jeremy, get off of him.

JEREMY
(*punching SGT. PEPPER one
more time*)
You don't ever talk to my friends like that! You got it!

TINY
Now, you assholes get away from my bus!

NARRATOR
HIPPIE helps SGT. PEPPER move to behind the bus.

HIPPIE
We didn't know, man. I mean -- we thought --.

TINY
You take another step and I'll put your ass on that bus! That what you want?

BOBBY MAC
(*through the window*)
C'mon, you long-haired assholes! Get on the bus. We'll give you a ride you won't forget!

SKI
Open dthe door! Don't dcall me a babykeeler, you modorfowkers!

EARL RAY
Get over here! I'll gouge your fucking eyes out!

TINY (*shouting*)
I said get the fuck out of here!

SGT. PEPPER
We're sssssorry, man. We didn't mmmmean no harm. We're sssssorry, man. We didn't mmmmean no harm.

TINY
Well, we did! Now get the hell out of my sight!

NARRATOR
TINY, MOOSE and JEREMY get back on the bus to cheering from everyone else. As TINY takes his seat, he smiles broadly.

TINY
This is going to be an exceptional trip.

> *Lights fade and go out,
> one at a time, stage right
> to stage left.*

ACT II

SCENE 7

SETTING: *FOR NINE-ACTOR READERS THEATER CASTING AND SEATING CHART, SEE PAGE 3. For both acts, all scenes: nine seats are in a row from left to right. If six wheelchairs are available, they should be used for seats 1,2,3 and 7,8,9. The center three seats (4,5,6) should be chairs or stools. The NARRATOR sits off the stage, at either side. In front of each seat is a stand holding a copy of the script.*

If costumes are available, MOOSE, BIG AL, SKI, and BOBBY MAC are wearing non-dress khaki uniforms, TINY is wearing US Navy Corpsman first class whites, and JEREMY is wearing his US Navy everyday whites. DAVE is looking fine in a three piece suit, and the ESCORT is dressed seductively.

AT RISE: *From stage left to stage right, seated are: MOOSE, BIG AL, EARL RAY, TINY, ESCORT, DAVE, SKI, JEREMY, and BOBBY MAC.*

NARRATOR
The MARINES and JEREMY have made it to Atlantic City, just in time for the Miss America pageant. Before the lights come up, out of the dark an announcer's voice booms into the void.

"Ladies and gentlemen. It is my great pleasure and honor to welcome our special guests this evening. Please join me in giving a big round of applause for the group of Vietnam Veterans from the U.-S. Naval Hospital in Philadelphia! We are thankful for their service and their individual sacrifices. Welcome, veterans, to the Miss America Pageant, and thank you!"

As the audience bursts into applause, the lights come up, one at a time, stage right to stage left. The patients and TINY are all sitting around tables in a high-class lounge, while DAVE and an ESCORT watch them from across the room. On the stage, Sitting in a row from the audience's left to right, are: BOBBY MAC, JEREMY, SKI, DAVE, ESCORT, TINY, EARL RAY, BIG AL, and MOOSE.

EARL RAY
What the fuck kind of name is Reg Morgan for a bar?

BIG AL
Hey, the guy at the pageant said this is a great place. It's gotta be better than that beauty contest. Anyway, they can call it Hell for all I care. Just get me a beer.

DAVE
(coming to their table and sitting on the empty stool)
Hey, ain't you guys the veterans that were at the beauty pageant tonight? The ones in the spotlights?

MOOSE
Yeah, that's us.

DAVE
You guys are the ones who've been to Vietnam? You're over in Philly, right?

MOOSE
Yeah, that's us. You're not looking for trouble are you?

DAVE
Hell no. This is your lucky night. The name's Dave Marzetti. I own this bar. Tonight, you guys help yourselves. Tonight, the bar's all yours. And you ain't going to pay a dime. Just ask for whatever you want. What'll you have?

SKI
Scotch and soda.

DAVE
What the hell. You don't need someone to mix your drinks for you. You guys can just mix your own. You don't need anyone else to do this. All you need is the booze.

NARRATOR
Dave waves at ESCORT, who brings over glasses and bottles of gin, vodka, whiskey and scotch along with mixers.

DAVE
You guys got everything you need? Anything you want, just ask for it. I'll get someone to get it for you.

SKI
(with a sly grin)
Well, dwe could always use a woman or two.

DAVE
(smiling and putting his arm around Ski)
I should have known. Just give me a minute.
(walks behind the screen)

BIG AL
Who's the scary looking guy following Dave around?

BOBBY MAC
It's Dave's bodyguard, would be my guess.

BIG AL
What does he need a bodyguard for?

BOBBY MAC
Because he does shit other people don't like, that's why.

BIG AL
What kinda things?

MOOSE
What's it fuckin' matter? He's doin' right by us, isn't he?

BIG AL
Hell, yeah!

NARRATOR
Dave has a word with ESCORT and then comes back to their table, bringing ESCORT with him.

DAVE
Come on you guys! We have a special room in the back for our special friends, if you know what I mean. My friend here is going to take each of you for a ride! And I mean a ride!

ESCORT
Come with me, gentlemen. Which of you handsome men wants to go first?

NARRATOR
The patients and TINY all look at each other, then back to the ESCORT.

DAVE
What are you waiting for?

MOOSE
That's all the encouragement I need.

BOBBY MAC
Oh shit, we don't need privacy! I'm going to watch. Been so long I think I forgot how!

NARRATOR
MOOSE and BOBBY MAC leave with ESCORT and follow her behind the screen.

EARL RAY
Just like the choppers in Nam, this is the jump seat. Even for you, Shoff.

JEREMY
(*holding up a drink*)
I'll drink to that!

                              BIG AL
Shoff, you're _my_ jump seat. Be ready when I am!

                              JEREMY
Alright, Big Al. This chopper's gonna fly.

                              DAVE
Next?

                              BIG AL
Get me in there, Shoff!

                              NARRATOR
JEREMY pushes BIG AL in his wheelchair behind the screen as MOOSE
and BOBBY MAC come out smiling.

                              JEREMY
                       (*returning to his seat*)
How about you, Earl? You ready to jump?

                              EARL RAY
You go ahead, Shoff.

                              JEREMY
You go, Earl. I'll get my turn.

                              EARL RAY
                       (*looking at the floor*)
No, you go, Shoff. I don't think I can do it.

                              BOBBY MAC
Sure you can, Earl. Just lay down and let her do the rest!

                              EARL RAY
It's not that, man. It's Jennifer.

                              JEREMY
Okay, I'll jump next!

                              SKI
Don't forget dme. I weel go next!

                              TINY
Not me! I know they'll make anyone who takes a turn get tested
tomorrow.

                              EARL RAY
You better hope none of you bastards have the clap.

                              BIG AL
Too late now! I still got the fungus from Nam!

                    BOBBY MAC
If you still got that shit from Nam, your dick would've fallen
off by now!

                    NARRATOR
ESCORT comes back out, assisting BIG AL in his wheelchair.

                    BIG AL
Yeah, well go ask the blonde about my dick.

                    SKI
My deek better not fall off. I dwill keek what's left of your
ass!

                    NARRATOR
ESCORT leads JEREMY and SKI to the back room.

                    MOOSE
Everybody who wants one get at least one jump?

                    BIG AL
Two for me!

                    TINY
Hey guys, it's almost five in the morning. We better get back.

                    DAVE
How would you guys like a little breakfast? I know where there's
a great buffet.

                    TINY
Thanks, Dave, but we really need to get back as soon as Jeremy
and Ski come out. If we don't get back soon, they'll put us down
as AWOL.

                    DAVE
Okay, but I'm getting your cabs back to your hotel. Here's a
business card for each one of you. If you're ever in Atlantic
City, call me. And if you ever are here and <u>don't</u> call me, I'll
know.

                    NARRATOR
JEREMY and SKI come back out from behind the screen.

                    TINY
On behalf of all of us, thank you, Dave! It has been an
outstanding night!

                    DAVE
Any time, men. Any time. It's been an honor.

                    NARRATOR
All the men shake hands and say their goodbyes.
                         (MORE)

NARRATOR (CONT'D)
As they head towards the door, TINY points to MOOSE, BIG AL, SKI, BOBBY MAC, and JEREMY.

TINY
You, you, you, you and you! All of you but Earl Ray are going with me down to sick bay tomorrow. That little episode has earned you a reward. You're all getting squeezed for V.-D.

JEREMY
What's he mean, squeezed?

BOBBY MAC
It ain't really squeezed, it's more like poked.

ROGER
The fickle finger of fate.

SKI
Dright up dthe old pooper.

MOOSE
No big deal! Just bend over and enjoy it.

NARRATOR
The men are all laughing and staggering as they go off the stage, with their arms around each other's shoulders.

*Lights fade and go out,
one at a time, stage right
to stage left.*

ACT II

SCENE 8

SETTING: *FOR NINE-ACTOR READERS THEATER CASTING AND SEATING CHART, SEE PAGE 3. For both acts, all scenes: nine seats are in a row from left to right. If six wheelchairs are available, they should be used for seats 1,2,3 and 7,8,9. The center three seats (4,5,6) should be chairs or stools. The NARRATOR sits off the stage, at either side. In front of each seat is a stand holding a copy of the script.*

If costumes are available, during the second act MOOSE, BIG AL, EARL RAY, SKI, and BOBBY MAC wear USMC uniforms. JEREMY, TINY, and DR. DONNOLLY wear US Navy uniforms; PAPPY wears a US Coast Guard uniform. In this scene, MOOSE, BIG AL, SKI, and BOBBY MAC are wearing non-dress khaki uniforms. EARL RAY is wearing his full dress blues, with medals and ribbons. JEREMY is wearing his US Navy everyday whites.

AT RISE: *From stage left to stage right, seated are: MOOSE, BIG AL, EARL RAY, DR. DONNOLLY, empty, empty, SKI, JEREMY, and BOBBY MAC.*

NARRATOR

In an arc across rehab Ward Q, from the audience's left to right, are: three empty wheelchairs, three empty stools with footlockers between them, EARL RAY wearing his full Marine Corps dress blues uniform with medals and ribbons, and two more empty wheelchairs. On the footlocker next to EARL RAY, there are a bottle of Jack Daniels and a small box. EARL RAY is holding a bottle of pills. As the lights come up, JEREMY, MOOSE, BIG AL, BOBBY MAC, and SKI come in, talking loudly. When they see EARL RAY, they all fall silent.

MOOSE

What's up, Earl?

EARL RAY

The sky.

MOOSE

You know what I mean. C'mon, what's going on?

EARL RAY

Just let it happen. Don't call for help until you're certain it's too late. Keep your promise. I'm feeling really lucky today.

NARRATOR

Moose picks up the bottle of pills.

MOOSE

How many did you take?

EARL RAY
Not enough.

MOOSE
How did you get so many, Earl? That's twice what they give you at the pharmacy.

EARL RAY
Shit, Moose, I can get twenty of these for a pack of smokes.

MOOSE
How many did you take, my friend?

EARL RAY
Four -- maybe five. I'm not sure. Probably not enough.

MOOSE
Then let's call it quits for now. What do you say?

EARL RAY
Just let it happen this time. You guys promised.

MOOSE
Don't let this be the last thing you do with your life, Earl.

EARL RAY
It's not, Moose. The last thing I did with my life was step on a land mine.

BIG AL
Jesus, Earl. Think about it for a while, huh?

EARL RAY
Shit, Al. You know damn well I've <u>been</u> thinking about it. I've been thinking about it for a long time, for Christ's sake. Don't stop me. Just stay close by. That's all I ask.

SKI
I dknow we promised, Earl. Eef eet's what dyou want weel be here. But, I'm asking you to not to do eet.

JEREMY
(*blurts out*)
I've changed my mind, Earl! I'm going for help.

EARL RAY
You can't, god dammit. You made a promise. All of you.

MOOSE
(*picking up the bottle of Jack*)
Let me have a drink of the Jack. Okay, Earl? Why don't you give me the pills, too.

EARL RAY

Can't do it, Moose. Even if I don't do it now, I'll need these when the time comes. But like I said, I'm feeling really lucky.

NARRATOR

As EARL RAY's friends stood gathered round him, a phone could be heard ringing from out in the hallway. Ringing. Ringing. It wouldn't stop. Finally someone answered it, and a few seconds later a VOICE could be heard yelling that there was a girl on the phone who wanted to talk to an EARL RAY. She said her name was Jennifer, and that she was calling from the front gate.

JEREMY

You stay here and I'll bring you the phone, Earl. The cord is long enough to reach in here.

NARRATOR

JEREMY goes behind the screen and returns carrying a rotary-dial phone, which he holds as he hands the handset to EARL RAY.

EARL RAY
(into phone)
Is this some kind of a fucking joke!
(pause)
Who is this really?
(pause)
Jen? Is it really you?
(pause)
Jen. Jen, it's really you?
(pause)
You're <u>where</u>? You're at the front gate <u>here</u>? At the hospital?
(pause)
What are you doing here?
(pause)
You want to take me home? Now? You're taking me <u>home</u>?
(weeping)
Oh, Babe. Oh, Babe. Yes. I'll go with you. I'll get the guys to help me and I'll be right down.
(Hangs up phone and hands it back to JEREMY. Looks up at MOOSE.)
I'm going home, guys. I'm going home.

NARRATOR

All the patients cheer loudly. They are laughing, celebrating, and slapping each other on the backs as DR. DONNOLLY enters the ward and slowly walks over to them.

BOBBY MAC

Dr. Donnolly. What's wrong? What are you doing out here?

EARL RAY

You look terrible. It's no fucking good, is it?

II-8-97

                    DR. DONNOLLY

No it's not, Earl. I thought it would be best if you guys heard it from me.

                    BIG AL

What could be that bad?

                    DR. DONNOLLY (*choking up*)

I'm sorry to have to tell you this, but Doc Miller was killed in Viet Nam.

                    NARRATOR

The patients stop, stunned, and look back and forth from DR. DONNOLLY to each other. No one speaks. All at once, the stage goes dark.

            PLEASE NOTE: This is the
            only scene in the entire
            play for which all the
            lights go out at the same
            time.

ACT II

SCENE 9

SETTING: *FOR NINE-ACTOR READERS THEATER CASTING AND SEATING CHART, SEE PAGE 3. For both acts, all scenes: nine seats are in a row from left to right. If six wheelchairs are available, they should be used for seats 1,2,3 and 7,8,9. The center three seats (4,5,6) should be chairs or stools. The NARRATOR sits off the stage, at either side. In front of each seat is a stand holding a copy of the script.*

If costumes are available, MOOSE, BIG AL, SKI, and BOBBY MAC wear USMC uniforms. JEREMY wears a US Navy uniform; EVA (seat 5) wears a silky robe over her hotpants. BAR PATRON (seat 6) wears a puffy, insulated vest over his dark pants and an open necked shirt.

AT RISE: *From stage left to stage right, seated are: MOOSE, BIG AL, empty, empty, EVA, BAR PATRON, SKI, JEREMY, BOBBY MAC.*

NARRATOR
Three bar-height tables with three chairs behind each one are arranged left to right at the Rainbow Bar and Grill. EVA and a BAR PATRON are sitting at the table on the audience's right. As the lights come up on each seat in order, JEREMY, MOOSE, BIG AL, BOBBY MAC, and SKI enter the bar, with JEREMY carrying BIG AL on his back. The patients pull the two empty two tables together and sit behind them. EVA walks over and begins talking to to the group.

EVA
Hey guys. Where have you been for so long? Is my dancing that bad? And where's Earl Ray? I've missed him.

MOOSE
He's in Florida, soaking up some sun and some lovin'. Jennifer took him home. You should have seen him the day she pulled up to Q ward. First time we ever saw him smile. We miss him, too.

EVA
So what's the occasion for your coming back?

MOOSE
Shoff has news, and he wouldn't tell us till we got here.

BIG AL
Yeah. What's such a big deal you couldn't tell us on Q?

EVA
Let's hear it, Jeremy. You look like you're about to bust.

JEREMY
(*grinning*)
I couldn't be better!

BOBBY MAC
What are you so happy about? You getting out of here?

                              JEREMY
Yeah. I got my review board decision today.

                               SKI
Dyou are geeting out? Dyou are going home?

                            BOBBY MAC
Oh man, that's great!

                              JEREMY
No, guys, I ain't getting out. I got my orders, but they got me
fit for full duty. Gave me orders for an aircraft carrier. I'm
headed for Nam.

                             BIG AL
No way! They can't do that.

                              JEREMY
They've done it. That admiral I pissed off made sure the brass
here didn't forget. He got the review board to overrule Dr.
Donnolly. But it's no big deal. I owe you guys at least a trip
over there.

                             BIG AL
You don't owe us shit. You serious? The boat you're goin' on is
headed to Nam?

                              JEREMY
That's what they say.

                            BOBBY MAC
Now, ain't that some shit.

                              JEREMY
You guys know it don't mean shit to be on a boat near Nam.

                              MOOSE
Well, I'll be a son of a bitch.

                             BIG AL
They got you, didn't they?

                              JEREMY
That's what it's all about. They made sure that smart-ass remark
I made to the admiral stayed in my records. And my mother's phone
call to her congressman didn't help much either.

                               SKI
dWhat phone call? dWhat Congressman?

                            JEREMY
It wasn't much. I happened to mention to my mom what the admiral
had done and she wrote some congressman a letter. I got called
down by the legal dudes to explain why I was trying to ruin the
reputation of the hospital and the good doctors here. Something
about a possible congressional inquiry, too. I signed a couple
of forms and never heard shit after that.

                            BIG AL
Holy shit! Your ass is grass even on that boat!

                            JEREMY
They can fuck with me all they want. Don't mean shit.

                            MOOSE
Ain't no way you're gonna go. We'll talk to Dr. Donnolly.

                            JEREMY
He's already talked to the board. They don't give a shit what he
says. I don't think they'll even put his report in my file.

                            SKI
Shit, man, dthey got us all by dthe balls if they want.

                            BOBBY MAC
You just finding that out? Be glad you still got balls!

                            MOOSE
Let me guess. You're telling us here because this calls for a
party!

                            EVA
Got that right! And not just any old party. The Rainbow's gonna
do it big and do it right tonight! The beer's on the house
tonight. It'll be a party of which Earl Ray would be proud.

                            BIG AL
Sounds good to me! We need more beer.

                            NARRATOR
EVA nods at BAR PATRON, who brings four more pitchers of beer.

                            MOOSE
When you gotta report?

                            JEREMY
I got one week left here.

                            BOBBY MAC
Well ain't that some shit. Uncle Sam took a dump on Shoff and
we're here to wash him off! We're gonna need a lot of beer to get
rid of the stink.

EVA
Well, don't get any of it on my bar. What did you do, Jeremy, to deserve this?

SKI
He peesed off the big brass over a dyear ago and they didn't forget it.

EVA
Must have been serious if they held a grudge this long.

MOOSE
They don't forget shit. The higher-ups are protecting their own asses.

EVA
What is it exactly that you did?

BIG AL
He told the admiral to shove it!

EVA
An admiral? That was a crazy thing to do, Jeremy.

MOOSE
Crazy enough we made him an honorary Marine!

BOBBY MAC
An honorary Marine and by-God relative, too! Let's fucking celebrate!

JEREMY
(*lifting his beer*)
To Doc.

All present lift their glasses in a silent toast.

EVA
Say, you guys got quiet all of a sudden. What happened?

MOOSE
We were just saluting one of the best corpsman in the Navy.

BIG AL
(*raising his glass of beer*)
No, to the best corpsman in the Navy.

BOBBY MAC
Yeah, here's to Doc Miller.

EVA
Well, why didn't you bring him with you? Where is he?

MOOSE
He's not here.

EVA
You mean he was transferred?

MOOSE
No. He's gone. Vietnam.

EVA
When is he coming home? Do you know?

MOOSE
He ain't coming home. He didn't make it.

EVA
(*crying and walking away*)
I am so sorry. When is all of this <u>ever</u> going to stop?

SKI
What do dyou say we call eet a night?

BIG AL
Yeah, we may as well head back.

BAR PATRON
How about another round for you guys, before you go?

BOBBY MAC
Thanks, man, but we're going to call it a night.

MOOSE
I've been thinking, Shoff. Like I've been saying, ain't no way you're going to get on that boat.

JEREMY
Says who?

MOOSE
Says me. They can't fuck with you like that, so you ain't going.

JEREMY
How am I going to get out of it? I ain't going to Canada.

BOBBY MAC
You're damn right, you're not.

JEREMY
Then what do you plan to do? Hide me on Q?

MOOSE
Nope. We're going to break your legs. You can't leave here with two broken legs.

JEREMY (*gulping*)
Break my legs?

MOOSE
That's right. Been thinking about this all evening, Shoff. It wouldn't take much. Just a table ought'a do it.

JEREMY
How the hell we going to explain it?

MOOSE
Shit, we'll just tell them we got in a bar fight.

SKI
I don't dknow about theese. Just geeve eet a break.

BOBBY MAC
Ain't this some shit! Let me help you with that, Moose! Wish to hell I had thought of it.

MOOSE
Okay, Shoff, all you'll have to do is sit down and put your legs straight out. We'll take care of the rest.

SKI
dYou are serious?

BOBBY MAC
Serious as a fucking bad land mine!

BIG AL
C'mon. Ain't no way we can let those bastards get away with it.

JEREMY
Damn right. Go for it, Moose.

MOOSE
What do you think, Ski?

SKI
Okay, if eet's okay with dyou, Jeremy.

JEREMY
What have I got to lose?

NARRATOR
JEREMY stretches out his legs.

BOBBY MAC
You ready for this, Shoff?

SKI
An honorary dMarine is always ready!

BIG AL

Oh shit!

BOBBY MAC

On the count of three.

BIG AL

Oh, shit!

MOOSE

Ready?

NARRATOR

Moose lifts a table over his head.

MOOSE

One!

BIG AL

Oh, shit!

MOOSE

Two!

BIG AL

Oh shit!

EVA
(*comes running over*)

What the hell are you guys doing? Good God, you need to stop that! Are you trying to kill him?

BOBBY MAC

Hell no, we're saving his life!

NARRATOR

Moose drops the table.

MOOSE

Oh shit!

SKI

Sawnoffabeedtch! Look what dyou did dnow!

EVA

Good Grief! Stop all this craziness and just get back to the hospital! I'll call you a cab.

> *Lights fade and go out*
> *one at a time, stage right*
> *to stage left.*

ACT II

SCENE 10

SETTING: *FOR NINE-ACTOR READERS THEATER CASTING AND SEATING CHART, SEE PAGE 3. For both acts, all scenes: nine seats are in a row from left to right. If six wheelchairs are available, they should be used for seats 1,2,3 and 7,8,9. The center three seats (4,5,6) should be chairs or stools. The NARRATOR sits off the stage, at either side. In front of each seat is a stand holding a copy of the script.*

If costumes are available, during the second act MOOSE, BIG AL, EARL RAY, SKI, and BOBBY MAC wear USMC uniforms. JEREMY, TINY, and DR. DONNOLLY wear US Navy uniforms; PAPPY wears a US Coast Guard uniform.

AT RISE: *From stage left to stage right, seated are: MOOSE, BIG AL, an empty wheelchair, PAPPY, empty, empty, SKI, JEREMY, and BOBBY MAC.*

                  NARRATOR
In an arc across rehab Ward Q, from the audience's left to right, are: BOBBY MAC, JEREMY, and SKI in their wheelchairs, three empty stools with footlockers between them, an empty wheelchair, and BIG AL, and MOOSE in wheelchairs. Two prosthetic legs and an arm hang on the side of EARL RAY's old wheelchair. As the lights come up, JEREMY, in his full dress blues, is picking up his sea bag.

                  MOOSE
We can still do it, you know. It's not too late.

                  JEREMY
Yeah, but I'm sober now. Things look a little different than they did a week ago. Besides, it's a damn ship. It ain't like I'm going on a patrol boat.

                  MOOSE
            (*lifting his left arm stump*)
Tell me about it.

                  SKI
Yeah, at least dthey didn't screw dyou like dthat.

                  BOBBY MAC
They're good at screwing everybody. One way or the other.

                  NARRATOR
PAPPY, in his Coast Guard uniform, enters stage right.

                  MOOSE
Well, look here! Ain't this some shit! What the hell are you doing here?

BIG AL (*hopefully*)
Pappy? The limo is back?

PAPPY
I took an early out. Couldn't see driving all the way to Florida just to turn around and drive back here. I got two weeks until I'm discharged from the Coast Guard.

BOBBY MAC
Well, son of a bitch. Welcome back to Q, Pappy the Sailor! By God, welcome back!

BIG AL
(*rolls over to look outside*)
It's here! The most beautiful thing I've seen since Tammie.

PAPPY
I thought maybe I could make a beer run later on.

MOOSE
Better make it quick. Shoff here's just getting ready to leave us.

PAPPY
Where're you going, Shoff? You getting out?

JEREMY
No early out for me, Pappy. I have a flight in a couple of hours. Going to San Diego and then off to see the world.

MOOSE
He's on the brass' shit list big time. They're sending him to Nam on a carrier.

BOBBY MAC
Just make it back in one piece, you got that, Shoff?

JEREMY
How will guys you ever know? We'll probably never see each other again.

PAPPY
If you don't mind, Jeremy, it would be my pleasure to take you to the airport.

NARRATOR
Jeremy shakes hands with MOOSE and BOBBY MAC.

JEREMY
We better get going then. I don't want to hold up a beer run.

MOOSE

You're not too bad for a noncombat mother -- for an honorary Marine.

JEREMY (*laughing*)

Thank you, my friend. Thank you.

NARRATOR

JEREMY reaches down and shakes hands with SKI and then with BIG AL.

JEREMY

You take care, Big Al. Make sure Pappy here takes you to Rosie's place. All of you take care.

BIG AL

I feel like I'm losing my legs a second time.
    (*BIG AL looks heartbroken,*
    then bursts out with a
    grin.)
Hey, wait! I just remembered! Earl Ray left something I was supposed to read to you before you left!

NARRATOR

BIG AL pulls a crumpled sheet of paper out of his pocket and smoothes it out.

BIG AL

Earl Ray says:
    (*reading*)
"You're okay for a noncombat --"
    (*looks up and grins*)
Oh, no. Wait. That's not what this says. I'm sure that's what he <u>meant</u>, but what he <u>said</u> was, "for an honorary Marine."

JEREMY
    (*making air quotes*)
Thanks, "Earl."

BIG AL

"So promise me one thing, Shoff."

JEREMY

Anything you want, Earl.

BIG AL

"Get that tattoo."

    They all burst out
    laughing, hooting, and
    hollering.

JEREMY

You got it, Earl.

                        SKI
dYou are a lot like us, dyou know. Eet won't be the same around
here without you, my dfriend.

                        JEREMY
And I'll never be the same without you guys.

                        NARRATOR
JEREMY and PAPPY walk together toward stage right. When JEREMY
reaches the curtain, he puts down his sea bag, turns around, snaps
to attention, and salutes the MARINES on Q ward. They return the
salute. JEREMY makes a sharp about face, picks up his sea bag,
and exits through the curtain, glancing back at his friends one
last time.

>   *Lights fade and go out,*
>   *one at a time, stage right*
>   *to stage left.*

                    <u>END OF ACT II</u>

                        The End

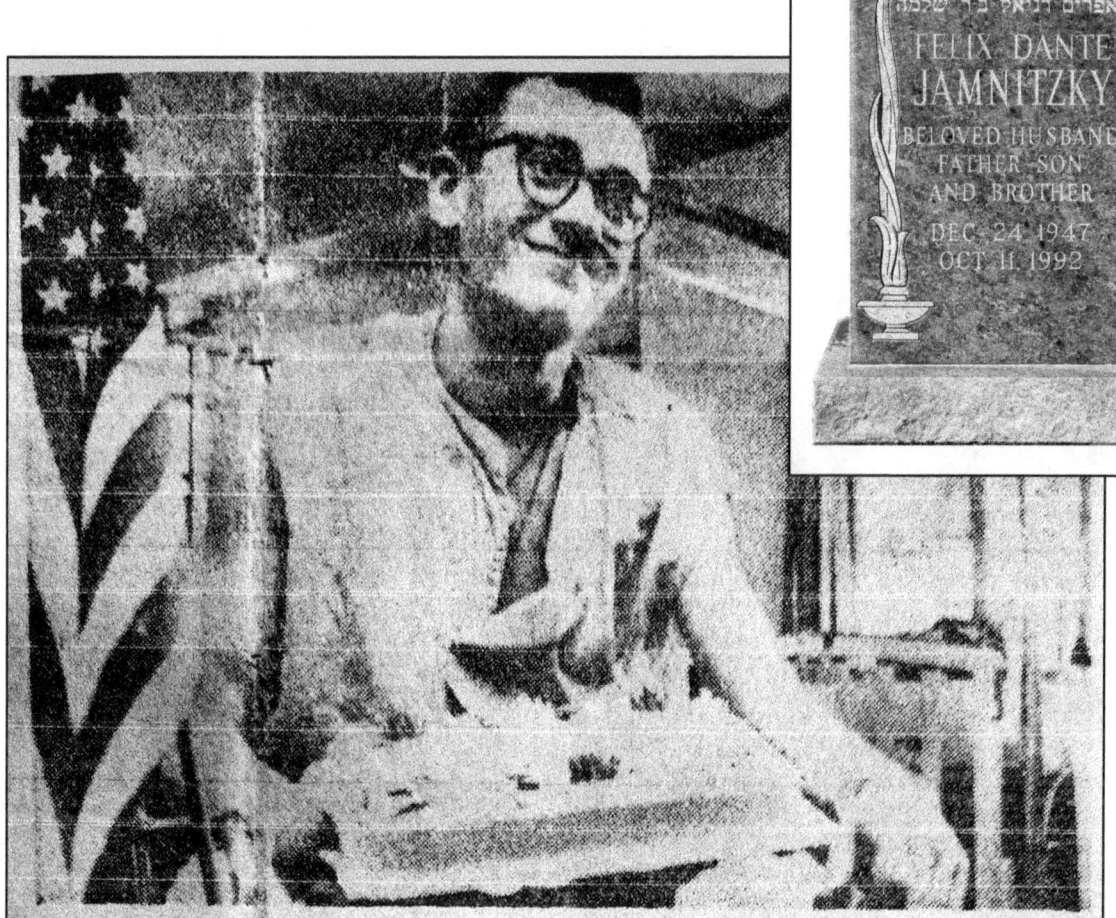

Marine Lance Cpl. Felix Jamnitzky, 21, a native of Argentina, sits in wheelchair at Philadelphia Naval Hospital after ceremony in which he became a United States citizen. He holds cake presented him by Federal District Judge John W. Lord Jr., who administered oath to new citizen.

Red Tape Cut in Hospital

DEDICATED TO THE MEMORY OF
FELIX DANTE JAMNITZKY

www.ingramcontent.com/pod-product-compliance
Lightning Source LLC
Chambersburg PA
CBHW080325170426
43193CB00017B/2908